Emotional Freedom Tec'
and Their H

T000621?

"The best on the subject! If you truly ⟨...⟩ ⟨...⟩ animal
companion toward wellness and create a harmonious household, Joan's
book is imperative. You'll learn how to do everything from breaking up
negative patterns to releasing the emotions and trauma causing challenging
behavior. Everything you need to know about EFT—and becoming the
guardian your animal needs you to be—is in these educational, informative,
and relatable pages."

—CYNDI DALE, author of *Energy Healing for Trauma, Stress & Chronic Illness*
and *The Subtle Body*

"*Emotional Freedom Technique for Animals and Their Humans* is something
every loving animal guardian should include in their library of essential
books—it's phenomenal, earth-shattering, brilliant, and groundbreaking.
Get the book, read it, and put it into action. You deserve it. Your animal
friends want it, and the world can rise if humans gain such knowledge!"

—Dr. RICHARD E. PALMQUIST, DVM, integrative veterinarian and past
president of the American Holistic Veterinary Medical Association

"Joan Ranquet gives the science behind the problems our animals experience while clearly giving solutions. Her clear charts and diagrams show the
specific points to be tapped on different species, with descriptions of the
physical and emotional indications for each point. Energy fields reach far
beyond our physical bodies and affect everyone around us. Your distress
about your pet's constant barking or nighttime feline howling magnifies
their imbalance and can make things worse. When you soothe both yourself
and your animal, miracles can happen."

—CHRISTINA CHAMBREAU, DVM, CVH, certified veterinary homeopath,
speaker, and author of *Healthy Animal's Journal*

"Joan explains the anatomy, physiology, and the reasons why EFT works.
The nerd in me loves all the details and explanations. The busy working
veterinarian in me loves the simplicity. Every animal lover, worker, and
dreamer should own this book."

—JILL TODD, DVM, certified veterinary acupuncturist, certified
veterinary chiropractor, and animal communicator

"Joan Ranquet's work with animals and humans brings deep compassion and self-healing to a higher level for all life. At first glance, this book is for animal companions. Glance again and find the healing tools for all humans—and all beings. Another great book by Joan!"

—MARGARET ANN LEMBO, aromatherapist, speaker, and author of
Animal Totems and the Gemstone Kingdom

"In *Emotional Freedom Technique for Animals and Their Humans,* Joan Ranquet provides a clear path to bringing the power of EFT to our animal friends. The book takes us on a journey through the development of EFT using shared stories, clear instructions, and fun exercises. As in life, Joan imbues her writing with compassion, humility, and wisdom. Each chapter brings us closer to understanding how our animals arrive at psychological disharmony in their lives and how we can be empowered to release the patterns holding them back from vibrant health. Anyone can learn and use this simple yet powerful technique to help their pets thrive."

—LOLA MICHELIN, LAMP, SAMP, founder and director of the
Northwest School of Animal Massage

Emotional **F**reedom **T**echnique for Animals
and Their Humans

Creating a Harmonious Relationship through Tapping

Joan Ranquet

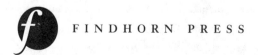
FINDHORN PRESS

Findhorn Press
One Park Street
Rochester, Vermont 05767
www.findhornpress.com

Findhorn Press is a division of Inner Traditions International

Disclaimer

The information in this book is given in good faith and is neither intended to diagnose any physical or mental condition nor to serve as a substitute for informed medical advice or care. Please contact your health professional for medical advice and treatment. Neither author nor publisher can be held liable by any person for any loss or damage whatsoever which may arise from the use of this book or any of the information therein.

Cataloging-in-Publication Data for this title is available from the Library of Congress

ISBN 978-1-64411-807-8 (print)
ISBN 978-1-64411-808-5 (ebook)

Printed and bound in the United States by Versa Press, Inc.

10 9 8 7 6 5 4 3 2 1

Edited by Nicky Leach
Illustrations by Becky MacPherson
Text design and layout by Damian Keenan
This book was typeset in Adobe Garamond Pro, Calluna Sans and Raleway
with Barlow Condensed used as a display typeface

To send correspondence to the author of this book, mail a first-class letter to the author c/o Inner Traditions • Bear & Company, One Park Street, Rochester, VT 05767, and we will forward the communication, or contact the author directly at **https://joanranquet.com**.

Contents

Foreword

Years ago, I had the pleasure of interviewing with Joan. Right away, I recognized her as someone significant in the world. Later, she asked me to lunch, but I couldn't meet her for quite some time because of my travel schedule and workload. Eventually, we met up and have been good friends ever since.

Aside from her sense of humor and wisdom, what I love best about Joan is that she has taken the trauma in her life and turned it into gifts. And then, she took her talents and opened a school to make other people's gifts shine. Joan is teaching people worldwide how to speak to animals, heal animals, and, most importantly, trust their intuition. I am so grateful for Joan and what she does daily for people and animals around the world.

Decades ago, I had a trauma on horseback that made me uncontrollably scared of horses. I loved horses, yet I was so nervous I did not want to be around them. I felt like a part of me had died, and I hated myself for it.

Joan offered to do the Emotional Freedom Technique with me. I didn't understand EFT at the time, but desperate to resolve this issue, I agreed. Surprisingly the tapping brought up a lot of repressed emotions, and I cried. It felt therapeutic to be seen for how much pain I was in, but other than that, I didn't give it a second thought.

Then, months later, I was at The Gentle Barn, Tennessee, with great confidence and joy, teaching my staff how to groom and lead the horses. My husband Jay, co-founder of The Gentle Barn, watched me do this and was confused as to why I was suddenly working with the horses after years of crippling fear. When he asked me about it, I realized that the tapping Joan had done with me had changed my life and brought me back to my love affair with horses!

Since then, I have trained with Joan to do EFT myself. I now do EFT for my animal communication clients, all of our animals at The Gentle Barn, and for people suffering from loss and trauma.

I've been rescuing and rehabilitating animals for over 30 years, taking in the most severely damaged ones with nowhere else to go. Time heals all wounds, but I always yearned for an easier, faster fix for their fear, heartache, and trauma, so that the animals I saved could suffer less and move on to their "happily ever after" sooner.

Joan and the Emotional Freedom Technique for animals she teaches allowed me to do just that for animals. This book will teach you how to do it! With clear how-to's, and illustrated through beautifully written stories, this book is an easy, delightful read that will give you valuable skills.

When I heard Joan was writing this book about tapping to teach people around the world to do it, I cried tears of happiness for the people and animals that will benefit from this remarkable technique and the beautiful way Joan writes about it. This book will change your life, your relationship with animals, and how you heal each other from trauma.

Enjoy!

Ellie Laks, founder of The Gentle Barn
www.gentlebarn.org

Introduction

I had always been the type to take a nap in a busy airport. If I needed sleep, there was nothing coming between us. I was first introduced to EFT because I had been the victim of a heinous crime and aside from injuries and PTSD to overcome, I was not able to sleep. I did this weird little technique called Emotional Freedom Technique, or EFT, with a hypnotherapist, and the next thing you know, I was able to sleep. And I am back to sleeping in random places if need be!

In the late 1980s, when I first started using animal communication, it brought such peace and joy to me that someone witnessed so completely the profound silent connection I had with another being. Finally, someone else was putting words to something I felt, and I knew to my core that my beloved horse, Pet One, experienced this same profound silent connection. I felt seen and my horse felt heard. It was truly magical.

Energy healing had that same sort of magical feeling. Sometimes the shifts were subtle and sometimes the shifts were remarkably obvious. Energy healing was both tangible and mystical, a very delicious combination. I love any place where it is quiet, vast, divinely connected, and full of possibility. That's how I feel when I'm with animals, nature, my creative space, and with people I love. Both animal communication and energy healing for animals elevate that space and possibility.

In 2002, when I was introduced to EFT because of my sleep issue, I had a very busy animal communication and energy healing practice. After years of private practice, in 1998, I started teaching animal communication and energy healing (scalar wave) and by 2002, I was teaching all over the country. I had a waiting list for clients. I was busy. I was like a kid in a candy shop. It was all fascinating, and everything was such an opportunity to serve and learn. Thanks to that hypnotherapist, through EFT, I was able to sleep again.

That prompted me to take a class, with the thought *Oh, the things I could clear on myself!* I recognized immediately the value of EFT for my clients and went on to get certified. I learned several more versions of EFT in the following years and got another certification in 2012 after a year-long program. In the beginning, I wasn't trying it on animals quite yet. You will hear in Chapter 1 how it came to be that I started trying it on animals in 2004! And there was no looking back.

In 2008, I started Communication with All Life University (CWALU), a program for people to learn animal communication or energy healing for animals or become a professional animal communicator and/or energy healer and commune with and advocate for nature and wildlife. EFT is a very big part of the school. As students go through the program, they get to help their own animals and have an incredible skill set to build an animal communication and/or energy healing practice.

Two other significant things happen. First, the people going through the program meet their tribe. They find like-minded people who have the same loves and passion and have probably never fit in completely elsewhere. Second, they go through a true soul's journey as they master these courses. EFT is a big part of the long and winding path. The more this work gets into the mainstream, the faster we could see more harmonious households. When a household has peace, it is as the acorn seed relates to the oak tree, a microcosm of what is possible in the world.

In all my years as an animal communicator and energy healer, the fastest path to shifting behavior has been EFT. The self-examination required for this work makes us accountable for our behavior with our animals. Through the investigation process of figuring out what to say as you tap (creating a script) on behalf of your animal, a true discovery happens about the animal. Sometimes, that moment of recognizing them creates a softness and compassion that truly starts the healing. You don't even have to be an animal communicator to do this. I have ready-made scripts in this book that ask the right questions!

I truly believe to my core that animal connection, communion, and communication are part of creating global peace. Being heard at a core level and seen for who we really are is one of the most healing things we can do with and for each other. If we all were to truly listen to animals, we would develop a deeper compassion for them and could start to share that compassion and listening with other animals—humans. We would see peace and compassion around the world.

After pouring my heart into this work and now this book, sharing stories dating back to the early 2000s, it's like I'm reliving all these experiences and am reignited by the idea that the possibilities are endless. I have worked with so many rescues, shelters, wildlife centers, therapeutic riding centers, guide dogs, emotional support animals, zoos, and, of course, private individuals to help move energy, create balance, shift behavior, bring healing about to health challenges and assist in a beautiful transition out of this world. EFT has been an essential part of all of the above.

As you embark upon the expedition this book will take you on, I encourage you to pack light and bring with you an ability to be quiet and listen. Even if you have never done any healing work and are doing this for your own animal, you are now stepping into the role of healer.

When I think of the profile of a healer, I think of someone who exudes healing. They don't have to do anything, say anything, and there's no Google. It is being rather than doing or knowing. A healer leans into discomfort and is totally comfortable being uncomfortable. While there, they don't do anything but hold space. By just being with the other being, no matter what technique or modality you use, you are offering them the greatest peace of all: an opportunity to be seen and heard. A healer is a fly on the wall that allows the other, the seeker, to experience their own possibilities with minimal guidance and/or facilitation. Sometimes, I think of healing as merely witnessing and celebrating.

I'm humbled and honored to share this journey of healing with you.

Part One
Fundamentals

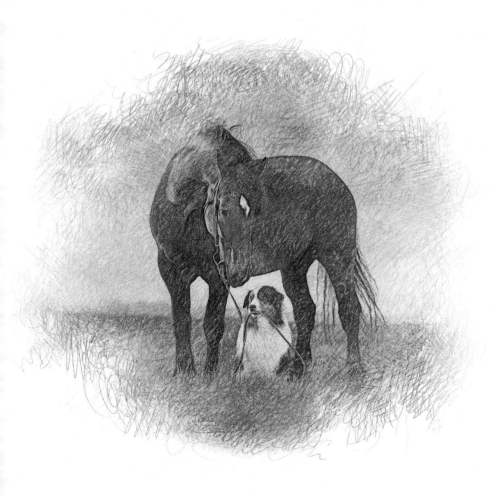

1

What Is EFT and Why Do
Our Animals Need It?

A human being is a part of the whole, called by us "Universe,"
a part limited in time and space. He experiences himself,
his thoughts and feeling as something separated from
the rest—a kind of optical delusion of his consciousness.
This delusion is a kind of prison for us, restricting us to our
personal desires and to affection for a few persons nearest
to us. Our task must be to free ourselves from this prison
by widening our circle of compassion to embrace all living
creatures and the whole nature in its beauty.

— Albert Einstein

Emotional Freedom Technique (EFT), aka "tapping," is an energy healing modality created by Gary Craig in the 1990s. Craig was inspired by Dr. Roger Callahan and his work with Eye Movement Desensitization and Reprocessing (EMDR), a technique used in psychotherapy to release trauma.

Fundamentally, the theory behind EMDR is that many feelings and experiences we have are the result of unprocessed emotions trapped or stored in the body. By using bilateral movement—for example, moving the eyes from side to side—you engage both sides of the brain (the left and right hemispheres) and the emotional processing needed to release trauma can begin. EMDR has a limitation, however: Only a licensed psychologist is authorized to do this work.

In creating EFT, Craig drew on the principles of brain science that underlie EMDR, making this healing technology accessible to all. Anyone can do EFT—including you! You'll learn the basics and more in this book, and will be able to immediately put Emotional Freedom Technique to work to bring relief and comfort to the animals in your life. And who knows? If you find yourself getting hooked on EFT like I did, you might even decide to pursue certification training in this powerful and flexible healing technique, one that has helped countless individuals, humans and animals alike.

The Practice in a Nutshell

To practice Emotional Freedom Technique, you lightly tap on a sequence of *acupressure points* on the body with the intention of releasing trapped emotions.

What are acupressure points, you ask? Let's do some time travel. Thousands of years ago, Traditional Chinese Medicine (TCM) discovered a system of *meridians,* or energetic pathways that run throughout the body. These meridians map to the physical systems of the body, and each has a specific theme.

There are 14 meridians in total, and 10 of them are associated with organs. Each of these organ-based meridians has a physical function as well as an associated emotion. Let's take the Lung Meridian as an example. In TCM, the lung is the main organ for the respiratory system, as you'd expect, but it is also connected to skin—or in an animal's case, the skin and/or coat. Emotionally, the lung is associated with grief. So tapping or acupressure on the Lung Meridian will shift energy connected to the breath, the skin/coat, and sadness or grief.

Each acupressure point has a very specific duty in healing the whole system: mentally, physically, and emotionally. And each acupressure point that has been chosen for EFT work has a specific purpose and potency. If you want to describe how EFT works in a single sentence, you could say this:

Emotional Freedom Technique releases triggering emotions through lightly tapping on "feel good" acupressure points.

When it comes to ways you can apply EFT to help your animals, there really is no end to its uses. The EFT healing method can quiet the nervous system while releasing old thought patterns that create fears, phobias, and anxiety. It can heal emotional wounds, as well as help alleviate physical pain. It is great for enhancing performance in the show ring, and it also helps animals in training and/or working environments slow down and focus.

The Heart of the Matter: Emotional Well-Being

Imagine that the body has great wisdom and the ability to heal itself, if it is set up properly to do it. This includes healing the emotions, which, as you'll soon learn, have a huge influence on animal (and human) behavior. Sometimes what we perceive as a behavioral challenge with our animal companion is actually something that is deeply rooted in emotional pain and/or trauma.

As an animal communicator and energy healer, I first started using EFT for the human side of the trauma that results from horseback riding accidents. Riders who have experienced an accident can hold tremendous fear about getting back in the saddle. That creates tension in the horse—you can't hide your fear from a horse—and the horse and rider wind up in a vicious cycle of mutual fear with no way out. In a circumstance like that, whether it takes one session or three or even more sessions, I have found that EFT is always worthwhile for the rider in bringing relief from difficult emotions.

An event like a riding accident generates more than just fear. Often, riders also experience:

- Loss/grief/sadness, because their situation has changed (sometimes dramatically).
- Anger toward themselves, because they failed to listen to their gut that day.
- Guilt, because they put their horse in a compromising situation.

When I work on a thorny problem like this, I listen to the rider describe the event and then have a communication session with the animal. That gives me a full perspective on all the feelings involved. From there, I can create a series of statements that address the emotions each is struggling with, to be recited while tapping the points.

When I first applied my knowledge of EFT to relationships between people and their animals, people with horses were an easy fit. Our working partnership with horses goes back millennia, and the emotional ties between horse and rider are strong. But then I realized that the same dynamic was at work for someone whose dog had been attacked by another dog, or whose dog had been the aggressor in a fight.

After an experience like that, when the human walks out the door with their dog on the leash, that person becomes ultra-vigilant. And then, just as happens with horse and rider, the dog picks up on that person's energy and instantaneously goes into fight-or-flight mode, alert for danger, too.

When I started listening to the person's side of the experience, I learned that they were experiencing, guess what:

- Loss/grief/sadness, because their situation has changed (sometimes dramatically).
- Anger toward themselves, because they failed to listen to their gut that day.
- Guilt, because they put their dog in a compromising situation.

And again, just as with the horses, I learned that the dog experienced a whole different set of emotions leading up to and following that same event.

My Shift to Tapping with Animals

In my early days with EFT, I only did tapping for the human side of the equation, and this actually worked very well, because when the person gained a sense of relief, ease, peace, or purpose, it changed the outcome for the animal, too.

Then, in 2004, in an urgent moment when I was fresh out of other tools, I started tapping directly on animals. I was floored by how well it worked! It all started with a horse named Shakespeare, and I'll share that story at the end of this chapter.

Because I had been doing energy healing for many years, when I made the jump to animals, I knew the signs to look for when a technique was working: animals releasing, relaxing, and letting go of their "stuff." I was amazed to see that the more I tapped on animals, the more release—and relief—I witnessed. It didn't matter what kind of animal I was working with: a horse, a bird, a dog, a cat. Not only did I see immediate results but I also saw sustained, long-term success, too. I watched, maybe a little mind-boggled at first, as horses started to have more confidence, cats quit fighting, dogs were more at ease with each other, and much, much more.

An Overview of Energy Healing

Now I want you to look at Emotional Freedom Technique through the wider lens of energy healing, because you need that big-picture view in order to understand what you're doing when you practice EFT. There is a basic truth at the heart of all energy healing transformation:

Everything in our world is made up of energy. Every living being, every form of life, is a force of energy. We humans—and the animals who are our traveling companions on this journey—are just that: energy.

The world around us is also made up of different forms of energy that create various forms of "power": chemical power, electrical power, heat, light, mechanical, nuclear, wind, solar, and hydro power, and more. Western medicine utilizes chemical power in the form of medications, and it also relies on surgery, a precisely targeted mechanical power. Western healing methods are also based in science, research, and deductive reasoning.

Energy healing, also called *energy medicine* or *vibrational medicine*, is different. It can be quite formal in its structure, or it may have no structure at all. It can even happen by accident! Because of its long history, this energetic or vibrational approach is sometimes called "traditional medicine."

The practice of acupuncture, which is over 6,000 years old, is a great example of a long tradition of energy healing. Many other healing or shamanistic rituals go back just as far and are steeped in the history of an indigenous people. The European settlers in the United States used a number of remedies—aka energy technologies—that are now considered "old wives' tales" but that actually worked and have withstood the test of time.

Energy healing is typically referred to as "complementary medicine" when the primary approach utilized is Western medicine. In this case, the energetic modality, technology, or technique "complements" this primary care.

Energy healing can entail anything from a complex series of practiced techniques to prayer, breath work, touch, dance, and the use of symbols, transmissions, activations, meditations, mantras, chants, and rituals. It includes using the energetic properties of substances found in nature as well, such as foods, herbs, flower essences, and essential oils.

Energy healing unites the body, mind, spirit, and emotions. And it allows for a "whole," holistic approach to healing at all of those levels of the person or animal. The effects can be subtle at first. Often after we employ energy healing, we won't know whether we achieved an actual "cure" for whatever the problem may be, but we can rest assured that there will be an impact on the core of the being who received the healing. And I can tell you this from experience: If you think of healing as something that moves through layers of stored trauma, some of those layers will be shed with each energy healing session, whether you are aware of it or not, and the healing will move to a deeper level with the next session.

Shifting Patterns

Most conditions, illnesses, and unwanted behaviors do not come on overnight; there is a repeated pattern at play. You can think of this pattern as a well-trodden trail. There are exceptions, of course, where the problem is immediate, such as ingesting something harmful or an accident and its resulting trauma. But even in those cases, a pattern created by the event will get reinforced through time. *Healing requires breaking up that patterning.* Often, Western medicine can set the person or animal in a new direction—surgery, for example, can quickly interrupt a pattern—but it doesn't necessarily create a new, healthy trail. Energy healing can do that, and it's one of its most important benefits.

The Role of Intention: Near and Far

Now, I have a question for you. What do you think is the one thing that all energy healing techniques have in common? It's *intention*. All healing modalities share a frequency—a broadcasting of a wavelength—and it can be fine-tuned by intention.

Touching on a point I made earlier, energy healing can take place "by accident" because intention lies at the base of all healing. You could be laying your hands on your dog while hoping it feels better (your intention), and pretty much no matter what you're doing with those hands, the effect will be healing, for both you and your dog.

Similarly, your prayer for the health of someone who lives across the globe is inherently healing. That's right, energy healing can take place when you're right beside a person or an animal and can touch them, but you don't need that physical proximity. You can be across the room or on the other side of the planet. In the same way, while EFT originated with physical tapping, it can be done at a distance as well. You don't have to believe this works—you can just try it. Importantly, animals don't have a belief system that questions whether or not EFT works; they just accept the intention and allow for the work to begin.

For close-up healing, you can think of one of the most famous healers of all: Jesus. He was a hands-on healer, touching the untouchable, reaching out with his own hands and miraculously healing the afflicted—spiritually, emotionally, and physically. Note that he also said, "Greater miracles than these *ye shall also do*." While we may not feel that we can heal at such a miraculous level, Jesus knew that healing was not the exclusive province of the gifted but something inherent in all of us, when it is coupled with the intention we all possess and can learn to activate.

In contrast to Jesus's hands-on approach, the first real known distance healing was documented in Traditional Chinese Medicine. If a doctor's patient happened to be the emperor, he was not even allowed in the room with him, especially if the emperor was very sick and therefore vulnerable. The doctor in that situation had to rely heavily on the emperor's attendant to follow his instructions. The doctor would indicate where to place an acupuncture needle (using that same meridian system I introduced you to earlier), which was attached to a fine thread and extended into the adjacent room where the doctor did his work. There, the doctor would sense the emperor's condition and conduct his healing through the feelings he received through the thread.

I share these examples of ancient hands-on and distant healing to point out that none of this is new. People across time have used their ability to sense energy and apply their intention for healing purposes. There is no reason *you* can't join this lineage, which we all share, and EFT gives you a very easy-to-learn technique that lets you become part of that ageless healing tradition—and give comfort and relief to the animals in your life.

Key to Energy Healing for Animals: Relaxation

EFT is among multiple methods you can use to perform energy healing for animals. I reviewed many others in my second book, *Energy Healing for Animals*. Many of these can be very relaxing for the animal and, in fact, can put it into a deep, deep sleep.

Sleep is so important for animals; indeed, for all of us. It relaxes the muscles and allows the body to calm down enough to allow the immune system to recharge. When animals' stress hormones are activated for too long, they can become more reactive, so it addresses that behavioral aspect as well.

Rest, relaxation, rejuvenation, and sleep also play a role in long-term health. Animals instinctively know this. I was once lucky enough to witness close up a beautiful example of this wisdom in action when I watched as a few guardian dolphins and orcas patrolled the perimeter of a large pod of dolphins, keeping their eyes and sonar alert to any dangers so the rest of the animals could dream in peace.

When healing is the intention, all energy healing methods can be employed to shift the energy and enhance the well-being of animals, as long as that all-important relaxation is taking place. Whether your intention is to heal a physical condition, emotional wound, or trauma or to shift an animal's behavior, relaxation must always be present.

A Tale of Two Nervous Systems

Getting to a level of profound relaxation not only helps rejuvenate and refresh the spirit; it actually goes deeper than that. It prompts the *parasympathetic nervous system* to kick in. The parasympathetic nervous system is also called the "rest and digest" system. It helps the brain calm down, signaling that danger has passed. And once the brain calms down, the body follows.

The parasympathetic nervous system also conserves energy so the body can use it to repair; it stimulates digestion and activates metabolism. We humans are lucky: We have the opportunity to intentionally make choices for ourselves every day that will shift us into parasympathetic activity and the experience of safety.

Our *sympathetic nervous system*—the "flight, fight, or freeze" system—is just the opposite. It telegraphs, *Uh-oh, uh-oh, uh-oh, danger!* And it's essential. It's what fuels our human ability to perform heroic feats like lifting a car off a baby—it gives us superpowers! When a wildebeest's sympathetic nervous system is activated, it has a shot at outrunning those stalking lions. With the all-powerful shot of energy the sympathetic nervous system provides, a mama bear can rescue her baby from a precarious perch on a waterfall and carry it to safety.

The sympathetic nervous system activates stress hormones, including adrenaline. This dilates the bronchial tubes so the lungs can breathe more deeply. It releases glucose to be converted into energy and pumps blood faster and harder for that life-or-death sprint across the Serengeti.

For us humans, adrenaline is great if we're preparing for a debate, a sporting event, or any other situation where kicking it into high gear is called for, but if the body doesn't have a way to calm down afterward, it comes at a price: that high-stakes adrenal explosion won't stop. The body will continue to experience increased heart rate and poor digestion, and as I'm sure you can imagine, over time this leads to disease and other adverse conditions. Emotionally, it results in anxiety, insomnia, and panic attacks, to name just a few such challenges.

Neither human nor animal can afford to live in a state of constant agitation, and this is something that is important to keep in mind, both for yourself and for the animal you are seeking to heal.

The Two Nervous Systems in the Wild

Whether predator or prey, an animal in the wild relies on a navigational system that is a combination of instinct, connection with others, and emotions. When the dominant predators in a woodland area are nowhere to be found, deer graze, rabbits hop, and birds sing, going about their daily activities—the parasympathetic system rules. But let a coyote show up on the scene, and the nervous system flips the switch: it's *on*! Birds sound the alarm and take flight, bunnies head for the brambles, deer vanish into the underbrush.

What exactly is that switch that jolts everyone into action? A single animal gets an inkling that something is up, and that awareness ripples through the *energetic ecosystem,* or, as Dr. Rupert Sheldrake calls it, the *morphic field.* That field of energy informs all creatures that are tuned in to it.

The energetic ecosystem extends to big predators as well. A pack of coyotes, a pride of lions, or a coalition of cheetahs operates within its own environment of energetic connection, or morphic resonance, in order to take down its prey.

Within the energetic ecosystem, herd, pack, pride, and flock animals are all used to taking their instructions from the leader of the group, whether mare or wolf. And many animals are in sync with other species as well. I've watched as the ravens near my home let everyone know that bald eagles are approaching, suddenly launching into what sounds like a screaming match. Everything within earshot knows what all that hollering means, and the next thing you know, when the eagles fly through, the world is utterly silent. Check back 15 minutes later, though, and robins, squirrels, and everyone else has turned back to doing what they do—rest and digest.

The same thing happens everywhere, as I have witnessed for myself as I've traveled the globe leading groups to observe animals in the wild. In many places in Africa, for example, springbok graze with zebra, giraffe, and wildebeest, and an invisible layer of connectivity among them protects them all.

Animals' lives depend on their ability to *track and react:* to continually sense the environment and react to changes in it. When it's quiet, the ecosystem they live in is a coherent field of energy. When a threat enters the scene, chaos ensues, and they resort to all available mechanisms for survival. When danger has passed, the collective energy returns to coherence.

Pressure and Release

Let's drop this down to the level of an individual animal. Let's say there is a lone duck on a pond, floating along by himself, minding his own business. Suddenly, in the distance through the trees, he sees two beady eyes staring out at him. A fox has fixated on our little duck—the duck is being hunted.

Our duck friend feels the *pressure* of being hunted, and his sympathetic nervous system kicks in. His body fills with the adrenaline that will prepare him for flight. He takes off like a shot. Then, while in flight, through the action of pumping his wings, the duck starts to *release* the adrenaline that has fueled his escape. Within just a few minutes, he lands on another pond. He beats his wings a few times, shaking off the remnants of the adrenaline jolt, and settles into the new environment. He sees his buddy there and paddles calmly toward him. The experience of fright has left his body—it was just a moment in time. He carries on, content to do his usual duck business.

This is how pressure/release works. The threat of the fox creates pressure, and the duck releases energy through the physical movement of flying as fast as he can. The entire ecosystem works in just this way. The herd of zebra grazing, their tails slightly waving in the breeze, realize that the coalition of cheetahs has surrounded them. That puts the pressure on, and the zebra speed away.

That's a dramatic example of pressure and release, but it's something that happens at a lot of different levels among animals. You can see it in action when the leader of a pack of dogs walks into the group. Responding to the pressure they feel from the presence of that dominant individual, some dogs won't even dare look at the leader. If the stallion or the lead mare in a herd of wild horses wants into the herd's shared space, everyone will move out of the way to make room. Their mere presence is the pressure the other horses need to comply with the established hierarchy of the herd.

Many methods of animal training make use of pressure and release, too. We ask for something by using slight pressure, and when the animal complies, the trainer releases the pressure and often offers a treat.

The Two Nervous Systems in Our Homes

This dance, this give and take between pressure and release, is how animals are designed to function. But what happens when animals are confined, kept in our homes and barns as we take charge of their day-to-day lives? In these settings, they don't always have the luxury of flight when they're under stress, yet they are exposed daily to things that add unnatural pressure to their world. Your doorbell rings. The neighbor's cat pees under the window, and your cat has no way to escape the smell. Maybe you have several species living together in your home that wouldn't normally share the same territory—now *that's* pressure. Maybe one of the animals you have brought into the home hasn't yet found its place or purpose in the family as a whole—more pressure.

Animals look to us for leadership, but look at us: We're living in a stressed-out world, feeling our own pressure over things like money, jobs, addictions, and more. Our animals perceive this chaotic energy— it's all too obvious to creatures that live not in their heads but in their senses. And they experience pressure.

When you look at this situation through that pressure/release lens, you can see how necessary exercise is in an animal's world. If they can't move their bodies, unlike our duck friend who gets to steadily pump adrenaline through his system one wing beat at a time, the animals we have chosen to love and to live with have no way of reaching the release stage.

To add salt to this wound, animals, of course, can't communicate what's going on with them in words—unless there's a good animal communicator handy. So the stress and pressure continually build up in their bodies. While humans have friends they can share their stories and problems with, therapists they can process with, animals have no such luxury. And so we circle back to Emotional Freedom Technique. Bodywork—*energetic bodywork,* especially; and EFT, in particular—can be essential in helping the animal we've brought into our world to heal and stay balanced.

Why EFT versus Other Energy Healing Techniques?

Emotional Freedom Technique is a form of energetic bodywork that cuts straight to the source of the energetic problem. As you tap on certain acupressure points with a specific intention in mind, the animal will experience release at multiple levels: in the mind, body, emotions, and spirit.

Over the course of an EFT session, you use what's called a "script," which offers an opportunity to break up old patterning. Basically, you tell the animal's old sad or hard story while tapping on feel-good points. This allows the animal to begin to release that old story and then, as you tap, to "install" or imprint a new, healthier story on the same points and channels. No other energy healing modality does this—and believe me, in my long career, I've used them all.

As with other energy healing techniques, with EFT you develop an intuition that tells you when to stop, when enough is enough. The script is simply a tool; it doesn't mean you won't also use your intuition to facilitate release. You can lean on the script to get you started, but eventually, intuition plays a big role.

Whether you are an animal communicator or not, you'll find that once you get into it, it's almost like you begin to channel the animal's experience. If you let go and allow yourself to "go for it," bits and pieces of information will pop out that you couldn't otherwise have accounted for. Tapping on behalf of the animal will give you deep insight into its inner life and what makes it tick.

Some of the revealed pieces you discover in the process are what I call the "tentacles": You learn that they are more far-reaching than you thought at first, and there are deeper layers to the story. Maybe the dog that was attacked by the neighbor dog had been attacked before, and you might want to tap for each of those distressing experiences as you learn about them. Conversely, you might discover that tapping with your focus on one attack releases all of them—past, present, and even future. Every situation, every animal is different, and you'll discover that for yourself.

I have many stories to share with you in this book to illustrate how EFT can impact the animals in your life, but let's start at the beginning with my first tapping experience with an animal, in 2004.

Shakespeare

First, my office phone started ringing off the hook. Then the home phone started chiming. A normal Tuesday meant that I had a full day of phone clients ahead of me, so when I saw on caller ID that it was my horse trainer, Chris, calling, I thought, *Surely, this can wait.*

But then the cell phone started blaring. I had only minutes before my first animal communication session was to begin. *Hmm, he sure is being persistent. Maybe this is an emergency.* I picked up the cell phone.

Chris blurted out: "Joan, you need to get out here to the show-grounds. Shakespeare is going after the ponies. He's going to kill them! You need to talk to him."

No formalities, no "Hi, how are you?" Just, *You need to get here—now!* The Chris I know is southern, low key, polite—nowhere near an alarmist type. It sounded serious.

At the time, I lived in Florida. The showgrounds were in Wellington, which was 30 minutes away. With my packed schedule, I would be lucky if I could sneak in an emergency phone session with Shakespeare, let alone drive out there to work with him in person. It just seemed impossible.

I suggested I could connect by phone in a bit, if I moved things around—I always tried to leave "wiggle" room for an emergency.

Then Chris stated explicitly what I'd heard in his tone: "You need to get here. It can't wait!"

The gravity of that plea finally got to me. I told him that I was on my way. Miraculously, it seemed, I was able to reschedule everybody else with a few quick calls, and off I went.

It was quite a scene that greeted me at the showgrounds. When I think of horses baring their teeth, I think of pterodactyls, and Shakespeare didn't disappoint. I even imagined wings as he menaced every pony that trotted close to his orbit. The little girls perched on their small steeds appeared stunned, like the terrified victims in a real-life horror movie.

Witnessing the scene, I was simply in shock, as was everyone else. I *knew* this horse—he wasn't like this at all. Where was this aggression coming from?

In my previous sessions with him, Shakespeare had espoused his love for his human, Karen, and respect for his trainer, Chris. He had a great work ethic and loved to jump. He was competitive, yes, but he could also be a homebody.

He liked the trail. He liked to vary the work he did, but he also liked some predictability in his schedule. He was quirky, yet proper without being stiff. He knew that today he was filling some big shoes for Karen; he had a job to do. He was a big-boned, stunning warmblood who talked as if he could show up in any warm-up arena, jump around it, then sit quietly before his jumping class and go in and win. In that "I can get this done" aspect, I'd call him a meat-and-potatoes sort of guy.

That was the Shakespeare I knew. In my previous sessions with him, there had been no hint of a pony fetish.

His person, Karen, is one of the most accomplished horsewomen on the planet. Beginning to follow her passion with her family on the race-track in the 1970s and then moving to the show ring, she was a lifelong horse person.

Shakespeare's trainer, Chris, is one of the most unflappable, masterful, confident riders I've ever known. He could jump through a ring of fire on a horse with thunder clapping above them and come out on the other side laughing and praising his horse. Like a true horseman, he adores his steed and takes no credit for himself.

But Chris couldn't control Shakespeare on that day. They would clear a jump and then, upon landing, Shakespeare would lurch forward—ears pinned, teeth bared like a rabid dog—toward any pony that happened to be on the other side of that jump. The little girls on top of the small horses would scream and canter off to safety (competently—they were strong enough to compete, after all) but clearly scared out of their wits.

Faced with this mayhem, I couldn't stop thinking about EFT. I thought: *I am going to try this. I have nothing to lose at this point. Someone could get hurt, or worse. I want to hear what Shakespeare has to say for himself in a session, but we need to employ something here right now, some kind of healing to shift the energy immediately.* I knew another technique, the scalar wave, would calm him, but it wouldn't change this behavioral pattern instantly so that he could function at a horse show. And come on—little girls were screaming!

I said to Chris and Karen: "I want to do something that is going to seem crazy, and it's going to look weird, too. We need to find a quiet barn aisle to work in, or else you need to not care what people think while you're poking at your face!" I ignored their baffled expressions.

We walked Shakespeare through what seemed to be a labyrinth of barn aisles until we found an empty one. I started with a quick communication session. Since I'd talked to him before, I knew his fabric—or so I thought. I wanted to bring him back to being *that* guy, *that* Shakespeare. Once we got quiet and connected, Shakespeare told me a powerful story that he'd never told me before:

In his youth, he had been weaned from his mother and sent off to live with some ponies— ponies that were mean to him. Though they were pony-sized, at the time he was very young and small in comparison, and he couldn't understand why they picked on him. Eventually, being a large breed, he grew—and grew—but these particular ponies never changed their attitude, and he was constantly menaced by them. That experience as a young horse had been terrifying. And now, all these years later and now weighing in at well over a thousand pounds of horse, he was still protecting himself from ponies. It still felt like life or death for him, and now he was putting others in that same situation.

I had done enough tapping with humans to know how to script an EFT session. Despite not knowing what I was doing in applying it to a horse at the time (I've created more of a system since then), I just jumped in.

I briefly showed everyone the points for EFT tapping. I tapped with my left hand on my own face while Chris and Karen imitated that. With my right hand, I tapped on Shakespeare's face and body. (You will see the points we used in upcoming chapters.) I had Chris and Karen repeat the scripting after me, and they tapped on themselves as well.

We started very simply, saying out loud, "Even though I hate ponies, I love and accept myself." *Tap, tap, tap.* We repeated that for a while, and then, as we tapped through the points, we released Shakespeare's old story of being bullied. It was a long and painful process. We went through his weaning and his feelings of loss from that, his hopes for friends and companionship with this herd of ponies, and his disappointment and other feelings related to having to survive after being threatened by ponies, instead.

Chris rode Shakespeare out in the warm-up ring later that afternoon. The horse was better around the ponies, and they got through the show. They even placed well, believe it or not. I thought that Shakespeare was tempted to revert to his aggressive behavior at points along the way, but he behaved himself well enough to pull it off.

A couple of years later, Shakespeare moved into a barn across the aisle from a pony and displayed no aggression toward it at all—this was the equivalent of achieving world peace! Eventually, when Shakespeare was retired, who was his retired next-door stall mate? A pony.

One round of tapping had relieved a lifetime of fear and aggression toward ponies. How could I not be hooked on EFT after that?

2

The Animal Worldview versus the Human Worldview

Usually—but not always—the more freedom you give an animal to act naturally, the better because normal behaviors evolved to satisfy the core emotions.

—Temple Grandin

When I asked who had an animal to tap on in class, Audrey volunteered. We were in the behavior week of Energy Healing for Animals, and let me tell you, when we resort to tapping in class, it's not because we're dealing with stellar behavior!

I asked Audrey what was going on. She shared that she was a caretaker for an elderly lady several days a week. The woman had three cats. One of the cats, James, was beating up on a more elderly cat. Not only was James younger but he was also bigger. In fact, he terrified both of the other cats, but only the oldest one would get injured on occasion.

I asked Audrey to describe how she would start the tapping if she were tapping for James. We were on Zoom, so she put James onscreen for all of us to see. She meekly tapped on his points and in a small voice (very unlike Audrey), tapped on his behalf:

- Inside the eye socket: "I don't mean to be bad."
- Outside the eye socket: "I don't mean to be bad."
- Under the eye: "I don't want to get in trouble."
- Top of the nose: "I don't want to get in trouble."
- Under the chin: "I'm a good cat."

"Hold on!" I said. "Stop!"

Audrey stared into the camera. I always keep the "*Hollywood Squares*" version of Zoom open, the one that shows all the individual images of the group side by side, one atop the other, so I can see all the other students' faces. Clearly, they were all dumbfounded that I had stopped Audrey when she was just getting started.

33

"Audrey, what happens when James beats up on the other cat?"

"He immediately gets put outside."

"Well, there you go. You're tapping from your perspective on what *you* think you would be thinking if you were a cat in this household. You're missing James's worldview. He sees it differently."

This is what we do in life with our own animals. We forget that we can have wildly different points of view.

So we backed up to the part where he gets put outside. And speaking of outside, I posed to Audrey this concept: "If you were a younger cat in a household with two older, established cats and a woman who is declining in health, wouldn't you feel like the outsider?"

Whether or not you do animal communication before you start a round of tapping on an animal, tapping for the animal means you truly have to look from their perspective.

Audrey understood where I was going from there.

I then said: "So, after he creates a bunch of commotion, in the end he gets put outside so he can romp and play and hunt, right? He's bored, and those other cats are boring."

"Here's what James is probably thinking, from his worldview: 'I'm bored. I feel left out. I want to do something. Crap, it's quiet in here! Certainly, these other cats want to play or something. If I can get the old one to scream, I can be put outside. Finally, I'll have some fun, for crying out loud!'"

Now Audrey had something to go on. She tapped with this intent, and as she did that, we knew James felt heard (which by itself will already start to shift the household) and felt included. Now he could be put outside before he caused a ruckus, *and* the humans could play with him, too, so that he felt included. Now, the household can reach a more harmonious tone. This is one of the many reasons I love tapping so much. Not only do we have to think outside of ourselves and truly see from the other perspective, but we are creating solutions immediately as we speak the script. When we get going with it, we step into the zone, and it's like we're channeling answers we couldn't have come up with before. They just fall out of our mouths in the tapping round.

In the case of Audrey and James, in a matter of moments, it was pretty clear how bored James was, and that meant Audrey could make a conscious effort to include him in the household and help him have more fun.

I'm a Good Cat

James wasn't thinking in terms of being a good cat or a bad cat; he was just being a cat named James. A cat isn't going to judge his behavior as good or bad. Instead, he'll create behaviors when he's around the other animals and the humans in the home based on getting what he wants.

He's discovered that if he's completely bored out of his mind, he can go pick on the other cat, the most vulnerable one. That cat will scream, and, *voilà!* The door to the backyard will open at the hands of whatever human happens to be around and doesn't want to hear the older cat being tormented.

If anything, James is a clever cat. He had figured out how to win the lottery.

We humans tend to be anthropocentric: We interpret the world according to our own human experiences. Another way to say it: When we interact with our animals, we make it all about us. We translate animals' actions according to our own experience, not bothering to try to understand theirs.

Operating from our own worldview, we expect them to think and behave in human terms, which, when you think about it, is impossible. This is why so many animals wind up in shelters. We think, *The way you're acting doesn't make sense to me. I don't get why you're not responding to me the way I would if (for example) somebody picked me up and put me outside every time I acted like you do. There must be something wrong with you.*

That doesn't mean that animals don't want to please or that they are trying to be "bad." They are perceiving their experience in the moment, according to their nature, and they have no sense of good or bad. That judgment is on us: we either like or dislike their behavior and then categorize it as good or bad.

If you are a dog out on an adventure and you happily roll in a dead animal carcass and then come home proudly wearing that, you aren't a bad dog the way you see it; you're a dog with the best smells ever! You now have the most coveted coat in town, and any dog worth their dander will be wondering where you got that smell. Meanwhile, we humans are horrified. *You stink! And why would you do such a gross thing? Bad dog! We don't want you in the car, on the couch, or even in the same area code until that stench comes off.*

If you are a horse that has plowed through the fence to join the other horses, you aren't thinking you are a bad horse; you feel triumphant! You're so smart for finally using your sheer might to knock down that fence. Meanwhile, your human's thinking probably involves cusswords and worries about how expensive or time consuming it will be to fix.

Each species has species-specific collective wisdom, instincts, bodily functions, and drives that can inform their behavior. Within species, the same thing applies: Each breed has breed-specific collective wisdom, instincts, bodily functions, and drives. And each individual has a blend of species and breed qualities *and* their individual, specific personality and soul that also inform their behavior.

In other words, we have to drill down on who this individual is *according to their own nature* in order to really help shift their behavior or create wellness from their genuine core. Even though Labrador retrievers were bred to dive into the icy waters of northeastern Canada to retrieve fish, there are plenty of Labs that don't like to swim. There are draft horses that were built to be steady, calm, and easygoing as they plow fields or pull logs down mountainsides, but yes, there are also draft horses that are just plain antsy. Most cats are prone to be moody, fickle, and standoffish, but you'll also find "dog-like" cats that want to answer the door, join the pack on walks, and ride in the car. Individuals don't always follow the guidelines that the species or breed archetypally offer us.

Then layer in the animal's previous experience interacting with humans. Sometimes the animal learned a certain way to do things in its prior home that is no longer relevant in yours, but they are entrenched in that behavior and aren't inclined to easily let go of it.

Sometimes, and especially when it comes to potty training, the animal simply doesn't understand what you're asking—in their world, it doesn't make sense. Or maybe they did at one point, but then they forgot. In neither of those scenarios do they think of themselves as "bad." That judgment of their behavior? That's you talking.

And Sometimes It's Just Fun to Bark

I will never forget the time I decided to spend the day barking with my dogs—or the expressions on their faces when I actually did it! My house is normally extremely quiet. At one time I was doing animal communication phone sessions or remote healing for about six hours a day. That evolved into teaching at Communication with All Life

University twice a day for up to two hours per class, three to four days a week, which I still do. And when I'm not doing that, I'm writing. So barking isn't just disruptive for me—it could kill my career!

I was living in Carnation, Washington, at the time. It was early fall and raining continually with no end in sight. That last high-pitched bark-fest between Olivia, Isabella, and the then puppy Delilah was like nails on a chalkboard. I couldn't take another minute. I wanted to storm out of the house and yell all kinds of cuss words, but I knew that wasn't going to be a long-term solution.

I lived on 23 acres, eight of which were open pasture, creating a mini valley where my horses could wander in the distance yet always be visible. My dogs were bark-crazy. They barked if a leaf fell, if a horse moved. They barked at seemingly nothing at all.

I got on my knees at the window and waited for the next round of barking. Sure enough, as far as I could tell, nothing happened to trigger it, but they started barking. So I started barking, too. They couldn't believe it. Now it was even more fun for them. And believe it or not, now I was having fun. Two great things came out of this:

1. Through barking with them, I found the on switch and the off switch, and now I can get them to stop quickly.
2. Human though I am, I learned how fun it is to just randomly bark at nothing; I highly recommend it.

If barking is that much fun, digging has got to be fun, shredding must be fun, scratching has to be fun, and on and on and on. (God knows, peeing on the carpet must be delightful!) So, you need to be aware that there may simply be a fun factor to an unwanted behavior. There could also be other reasons for continuing an activity, even after an animal has been reprimanded for it.

These are four common ones:

- They could be in pain.
- They could be overstimulated.
- In the case of horses, they could erupt in bad behavior if their equipment is wrong.
- They could be triggered by an old memory from their last household.

We Take Everything So Personally

Remember, an animal's superpower is instinct, and those instincts keep them in the moment in life. Our superpower is logic, and unfortunately when it comes to animals, it isn't always our greatest feature. That's because the logic we apply to animal behavior is based on our own worldview.

I bring this up at this point because our anthropocentricism often morphs into anthropomorphizing: interpreting animal behavior in terms of human characteristics. At its finest, we make up scenarios and belief systems about animals based on our own highly complex emotional lives. In other words, we take everything personally.

Years ago when I used to ride my horse Gabrielle and she would buck, I remember having the fleeting thought *Doesn't she know I'm a starving artist, and this is the only time I have, and we are absolutely doing this right now?* Not, *I wonder why she's bucking?* Or, *is the tack I put on her today in good working order?*

As I was starting to write this section, already knowing the answer, I asked around to see if any of my students ever took things their animals did personally.

Maria shared what she says to her dogs after they've peed in the house: "Don't you love me? I rescued you from a bad situation. Is this how you treat me? Don't you love your mother? What's wrong with you? I love you so much, I do everything for you, I work so hard, and this is what you give me?"

If I've heard it once, I've heard it a thousand times: "It's just not fun anymore to go on a walk," because a dog explodes in enthusiasm or yanks them on the leash. That frustration leads to resentment, and that leads to a sense of dread.

Then comes the negotiation. "Well if you didn't drag me down the road, we'd go more places." Or "If you didn't pee in the living room, you'd have more freedom." Or "If you weren't so herd-bound with the other horses, we'd go on more trail rides." This considered human logic meets in-the-moment, animal instinct, and no communication takes place at all. The animal–human relationship gets nowhere.

Animal communication and healing can't be about negotiation, much as your human self thinks you might be able to reason your way out of your animal troubles. They must be about deep listening, getting to the core of understanding *them,* and allowing the transformation of healing to take place from that standpoint. Understanding why the dog is dragging you down the street is the real question you need to find an answer to—*their* answer to the question, not yours. One option is to bring in an animal communicator to listen to the animal and break down the minute-by-minute factors that explain why your dog might go from exuberant puppy energy, excited by the jangle of the leash at the door, to nightmarish fang-bearer and a dog you don't even recognize anymore.

If there is no animal communicator in the picture, though, you can use EFT to get to the truth. The beauty of working with EFT is that even if you don't know what's going on with your seemingly crazed dog, you can *imagine* a "why" this might be happening, and you can *imagine* the emotions underlying the experience, and tap accordingly. And with some experimentation, the next thing you know, you are getting to the animal's worldview.

Getting to Neutral

"Oh, that horse is so sad," said a young woman as she looked upon a horse whose ribs were showing. The horse's face was hidden under a fly mask to protect her eyes. The young woman hadn't seen the horse or her expression before she made that statement. She drew that conclusion based on being able to see the ribs.

"What makes you say that?" I asked.

"Well, look at her, she's so skinny."

I took the opportunity to fill her in. "Well, this horse is anything but sad. Her name is Gabrielle. She's 34 years old (the woman gasped). She's been with me for over 28 of those years, and she had been my old boyfriend's horse prior, so I've known her 30 years. She's lived all around the country. After my divorce, she talked me into moving onto horse property and living with horses. She's talked me out of riding dressage with her—in fact, she talked me out of riding her, yet I still carted her around the country as my prized pony. And she pretty much tells those other two horses in the pasture here how to run their lives. This horse is anything but sad."

But we do that, don't we? We take what we see at face value and assume that we know how someone or something is feeling based on our own feelings, or our filters, or our past experience. The woman who met my old horses didn't know how difficult it is to keep weight on older horses, so she couldn't and didn't take that into account. She had no idea how many things Gabrielle had done or seen in her 34 years.

How can we finally see from the animal's perspective? When we can take our own feelings out of the way, we can be more *neutral* when we meet the animal where they are. And dare I say it? We can also be more compassionate. (Even as we still have to redo the floors because of bad potty training.)

In my animal communication and energy healing classes, we have ways to get to neutral. We have a standard meditation to unhook ourselves: physically, mentally, and emotionally.

EXERCISE

Take a few minutes to just breathe into the bottoms of your feet. With each breath, imagine you are letting go of any physical, mental, and emotional bits and pieces that stand in the way of your getting to a neutral space. Imagine that you are now completely neutral.

Why is this so important? Because we don't want our own experience to color that of someone else.

For example, if I had a horse that died of colic, if I'm not somewhat neutral, I will assume that any other horse I meet will die if they have colic; I will project that experience onto them. This is not helpful. If I understand that everything is energy, including my projection, it could do more damage than good. That is why my school subscribes to the philosophy "Healer, heal thyself."

A projection is a stuck form of energy—it is unhealed energy. If we are trying to help others, any baggage we have not worked through must be checked at the door; otherwise, we get caught in a kind of surreal luggage carousel that never stops going round and round and round. After a while, we don't know which baggage is ours and which is someone else's—it all starts looking and feeling the same.

If emotions are meant to flow (and they are), it is important to recognize your own feelings and do a self-check before helping another being so you can be clean and neutral. That's because, fundamentally, when an animal is in need of healing, you are basically walking into a situation where their own emotions aren't flowing.

Let's pretend for a moment that you are completely neutral. Now let's go through a list of things that would stand in the way of emotional flow for animals and their human companions. Throughout Part Two, as we go through the emotions and create scripts, you will see these limiting experiences at work as I illustrate them through stories of both people and animals.

Blue Ribbon Emotions

Reward-based training—also called positive reinforcement—is all the rage among trainers today. It is based on creating conditions for an animal to feel good and to be rewarded for what they are doing. After all, like people, animals want to feel good, right?

Put in terms of the pressure/release model, you ask an animal for something—that's the pressure—and then the release is the reward. Marc Bekoff and Temple Grandin reference "blue ribbon emotions" in their work. This excerpt from my book *Energy Healing for Animals* bears repeating:

> Dr. Jaak Panksepp, a neuroscientist and the author of *Affective Neuroscience: The Foundations of Human and Animal Emotions,* has a theory based on the "blue ribbon emotions" we share with animals. He writes that these shared core blue ribbon emotional systems "generate well-organized behavior sequences of the brain." In other words, you get the same behaviors when you stimulate the same areas over and over again.

Animals are not too unlike men; they seek safety, sex, and food. If we've spayed and neutered an animal, we've taken away the sex part. So then, what if it just comes down to safety and food? What is standing in the way of that? Often lots of things, especially for domesticated animals.

Temple Grandin, animal behaviorist (as well as spokesperson for autism issues), has linked with Panksepp's ideas on a basic list of blue ribbon emotions. According to both Panksepp and Grandin, animals' emotions are:

- SEEKING
- RAGE
- FEAR
- PANIC
- LUST
- CARE
- PLAY

Panksepp always capitalized these core emotions because they are that big and that primary. Of course, there are other emotions involved, which come after the initial blue ribbon emotion.

The same types of neural pathways and chemistry are found in approximately the same area of the brain in all mammals. Emotions play a key role in what motivates all beings. Emotions play a key role in decision making.

Dogs learn quickly to adapt to the concept that "If I sit and she praises me, that is good." And the next time the dog is asked to sit, they likely do. This emotion of feeling good creates a pattern of behavior.

If we were to subscribe to this simple list for both humans and animals, I think the world would be an easier place to navigate. As you will see throughout the next chapter and in Part Two of this book, there is actually more complexity than this list when it comes to humans—and at times for animals as well. But if we can keep it to this simple model when we use EFT to heal our animals, we will find that they move through their emotions relatively quickly and have decent breakthroughs each time—often well before the human involved manages to break through their own stuck energy.

If a human's blue ribbon emotions fail—that is, if we don't feel good about something we did—we will reflect upon the situation and try to come up with a different outcome in the future, based on our processing of the event. Animals, however, don't have the cognitive processing abilities that we have, and this may actually compound or entrench their behavior.

Brain chemicals associated with each of the primary blue ribbon emotions flow through the body and set off further behaviors and feelings:

- Seeking triggers dopamine by stimulating investigation, motivation, hope.
- Fear produces adrenaline and cortisol and creates a fight, flight, or freeze state. Long term, it can create anxiety.
- Rage kicks off the amygdala structure in the brain and produces adrenaline and cortisol. It can create snarling, aggression, and/or an actual fight.
- Panic also produces adrenaline and cortisol and can create grief and sadness.

- Lust is linked to the sex hormones, testosterone and estrogen, while attraction involves dopamine, serotonin, and norepinephrine. Well, need I say more?
- Care results from the production of oxytocin and natural opioids, or endorphins. These are the feelings of love and unconditional love.
- Play brings pure joy to the world via the release of feel-good endorphins.

That said, the benefits of certain behaviors can get in the way of healing or shifting an unwanted behavior in the household, both for the human and the animal. I will address each of these below.

Secondary Gain

A *secondary gain* is something new that an animal or a human gains based on the primary situation at hand. It can be something that is consciously pursued or an unconscious hidden agenda. Examples include:

- For the animal: James the cat getting to go outside is a secondary gain to being in trouble all the time. When an animal is sick or lame and they get a lot of attention, that can feel good and be a secondary gain based in a negative situation. In contrast, a stinky dog being dragged into the bathtub is *not* a secondary gain for the dog!
- For the human: The human may love the sympathy or the story involved with having a lame horse or a sick dog or a naughty cat.

Familiarity

When something feels familiar to an animal or a human, they can continually re-create it in everything they do. It could be familiar to:

- Be the leader.
- Turn every situation into chaos.
- Be taken care of.
- Be the hero.
- Have things be messy.
- Not get along well with others (including our animals).

And the list goes on and on. Examples include:

- For the animal: For James the aggressive cat, getting into trouble became familiar—just how his days always went. Other animals might find the caregiving they receive if they are lame or ill so familiar that they recreate their lameness or relapse into illness.
- For the human: Humans get used to having problems and sharing their boohoo story with all their friends—and anyone else who will sit still and listen. Meanwhile, their animal might be thinking, "It isn't *that* bad." A person who grows up in a chaotic environment may feel like having an out-of-control animal fits perfectly (even though it causes them anguish and they pay professionals to try to undo it).

Blocks, Resistance, and Battles

I put these three things together because they are pretty common and very closely related.

A *block* can be as simple as something that sometimes happens with my dog Abby. When Abby was young, she was in the hallway by the front door and the ironing board fell behind her. (If you know me, it's probably scaring you to think I even *have* an ironing board. But I do.) When the metal legs hit the tile floor, it startled her badly.

Ever since then, if she is in a narrow area and there is something behind her, she has a sketchy, tentative moment when she looks around behind her (God forbid even a plastic bag, floating to the floor). She has a block around the idea that she can safely walk through a narrow passageway. I have learned that I have to carry everything in front of her.

More Examples of Blocks

- Blocks can also happen physically. This is closely related to muscle memory. If an animal remembers being lame, they are blocked from putting their full weight on that limb. This is actually related to the impulse of avoiding pain in order to survive. If they think something is going to hurt, they won't move forward with a normal gait. Animals have more of an ability (and agenda) to mask pain. While these two things seem in contrast with each other, either can be true.

- Blocks for the human can be related to training. Another form of block is being unable to see a path to wellness in the current animal companion when the trauma of the last loss is still living inside the human's heart.

Examples of Resistance

Resistance can be that little voice in the head that says, *Nope. What if I fail?*

- For both humans and animals, resistance can show up in training.
- Resistance also shows up after an accident.

Examples of Battles

- People and animals both engage in battles. Some of us are very rebellious (speaking for some friends). Animals can seem to have what is often diagnosed in humans as ODD, or oppositional defiance disorder.
- If there has been a lot of trauma in an animal's past, battle may be the only path forward it can see. They head straight into the red zone, and there may be a fight to the death. It will be important to find the source of this and bring down that high emotion.
- Humans may have been taught that battling an animal is the only way to train it, because they had an old-school trainer. Or they may think it's the only way to "win" in a training situation, because they weren't effective in trying other techniques in the past.
- Some people and their animals have a battle as a bad habit. I am guilty as charged. I had a horse that had to have a giant battle with me before he got in the trailer. We "upped" each other's energy, meaning he would resist and then I would get stronger. He would resist more, and now some cuss words came out. This would go on for a long time. In the end, it was a very fun game for him. I think he knew he had me at the cuss words.

Beliefs, Vows, and Loyalties

Beliefs, vows, and loyalties are sensations and experiences that carry over from a human childhood, an animal's first household, or even from past lives—human and/or animal. And beliefs, vows, and loyalties often run deep.

Beliefs

Beliefs are an acceptance in the mind that something is real. It carries a confidence.

- An animal's belief is based on their lived experience: *The trailer is scary. Crates are confining. There's a bogeyman in my litter box.*
- Some human beliefs are: *I don't trust dogs; they all bite. I don't think cats are friendly, they can turn on you without any reason. Horses are terrifying.*

Vows

Vows are a solemn promise, of any kind, a pledge. Vows are very powerful.

- Animals that have been traumatized by humans will make a vow to prioritize their own safety at the expense of the human (the same can be true of feral animals). Sometimes it's as simple as *I will never trust a man wearing a hat.*
- A human might vow: *It was so painful to lose my last dog—I won't get another animal again. I will never let an animal suffer this way again. I will never go to that vet. I will never do that type of training again.*

Loyalties

Loyalties are very complex. A good example is not really recognizing how deeply wired we are by our parents' belief systems, yet remaining loyal to those feelings.

- Animals can feel loyalty toward anyone who loved them or anyone they have loved. Like children, they can even feel loyal to those who haven't treated them well.

- A human adopting a new animal might feel so loyal to a beloved animal that has passed that they think they've moved on "too soon."
- Sometimes the human will be so bereft over the loss of the beloved animal that they can't see or care for the other animals that are still alive in the household. In fact, they will often resent them.

Is This a Good Match Emotionally?

As humans, we love to wrap things up neatly and tie them with a bow. We adopt beliefs about what's going on with our animals that fit neatly into our own notions of what's going on (*My dog is mirroring me. My cat took on my disease*).

The truth is, they can reflect an aspect of us mentally, emotionally, physically, and spiritually, but they are still their own being.

I find the idea that animals are merely mirroring us not only egocentric but at the center of our anthropocentric consumerism here on Planet Earth—it is the ultimate "all about me." Thinking that they have created themselves in our image makes them "less than" us. It doesn't acknowledge them as souls in their own right, with their own stuff to work through (that may or may *not* be about us), with their own wounding, healing, karma, and trajectory.

Certainly, yes, you and your horse could both have a left leg injury at the same time. Maybe even from the same accident. You and your cat could both have kidney failure. You and your dog could both be dealing with aggression.

But how each of you got there is the path we want to explore—driving back to the beginning, for each of you. And at that point, you may find how many emotions you do and do not share, and how the ones you don't have in common could be compounding a bad situation.

For example: Let's say you and your dog have allergies. The dog has a suppressed immune system and is tightly wound. You have a suppressed immune system and are tightly wound. Your dog may be "taking on" your symptoms but doesn't feel responsible for *your* allergies. But once you establish you both have this same challenge, you could have an additional set of feelings that are contributing to the animal's sense of being tightly wound. You might have guilt, sadness, helplessness, agitation, or frustration that you've "given" your allergies to your dog.

In fact, every time the dog goes to scratch their ears, instead of gently taking the paw away from the ear, you might snap and say, "Leave it!" This could wind you up even more, and ultimately the dog senses that pressure—and, guess what, winds up tighter, too.

You as the human may often feel more linked to this animal with the same set of challenges, and it also may lead to deeper frustration for both of your conditions. And, again, how you each got there is a vastly different story. And those are the sorts of things we investigate as we create the script.

3

The Script

Some people talk to animals. Not many listen, though.
That's the problem.

— A.A. Milne

I would be so rich right now if I had a dime for every time I've heard "I would love to try tapping, but I don't know where to start." My other potential wealth-increasing statement would be, "How do I know what to say when I'm tapping?"

Worry not. For those of you who are new to this whole experience and don't know what to say or where to start, or what a script is, it can seem a little overwhelming, so let me explain.

By *script,* I am referring to the words that are said during the actual tapping sequence. The script starts with a lot of investigative questions, and I have laid them all out for you. I have created a sample script in this chapter with all of my investigative questions for both the human and the animal. Part Two is full of sample scripts and lots of stories. We are creating a script based on an experience that both the animal and their human are having in the present moment. This script could be created because:

- Both the animal and their human are having a bad experience based on a trauma they shared.
- The animal is triggered by a past experience.
- The human is triggered by a past experience.
- The relationship between the human and the animal isn't deepening.
- The relationship between animals in the household really stinks.
- The animal is exhibiting emotional overwhelm such as anxiety, aggression, timidity, all-out fear.
- The animal is exhibiting behavioral expressions that are unwarranted or unwanted.
- The human is going through something and the animals in the household are experiencing fallout.

Those are just a few examples of what could create a story. Scripts are based on stories, including EFT scripts.

But more than stories, Emotional Freedom Technique or tapping scripts are based on the feelings that are fueling the stories. So depending on the scenario, in Part Two, I have created investigative questions that lead you right into the "script," and like a little fledgling, you can fill out those forms based on the challenge and jump out of the nest and tap away!

Another definition of script is "plan of action." Literally, the tapping investigative questions that form the script create a plan. The beginning is more of the story, the middle is more of the emotions, and the end has a transition into what we want the future to look like. In some ways, part of the magic of this technique is that you are able to anchor in or imprint into these feel-good acupressure points the exact outcome you and/or your animal desires. Just as a side note, animal communication makes this whole "script thing" easier!

Beginning, Middle, and End

Every script has a beginning, middle, and end, just as every story does, and within that script, there are transitions. But I'm getting way ahead of myself here. Let's just start with the basics: getting an overview and finding the beginning.

I like to ask a lot of questions. I get my information from the human by asking questions about their experience and the feelings they have had and continue to have about the experience. I get my information from the animal through either the animal communication session or asking their human "What do we think your animal *feels* about this?"

Don't worry. I've set up these scripts in the upcoming chapters for people who don't even do animal communication.

When I walk into a situation (walk into a home, a barn, get on a Zoom or an old-fashioned phone call), I get a big overview from the human.

Let's take the Audrey and the cat story from Chapter 2.

The cat, James, is always in trouble. He lives in a household of elderly beings (overview) that don't want a lot of disruption. James is bored. He needs stimulation (James's specific motivation), and he entertains himself and gets what he wants by being naughty. Deep down, James, like anyone else, would love to be adored, but he's in a big pattern now that he can't get out of. James's tragic flaw is that he isn't seen for who he is and gets blamed for everything.

The beginning of the script sets up the story, what you are actually tapping about. The middle of the script is usually what I refer to as the "vegan sandwich meat": It is full of big emotions with lots of twists and turns, like a good plot, or it is one straight emotion of the animal if they aren't budging emotionally. The end is what I call "In a perfect world...": the projection/visualization of what we all want.

Remember this is Emotional Freedom Technique not "great script freedom technique." You don't have to have some perfectly crafted script before you begin. Having a sense of what happened and the feelings/emotions still connected to the situation are all you need to help the animal (and their human) release the pattern.

What Are Transitions?

In order to go from the beginning to the middle to the end, there are transitions. A *transition* in a story is an idea or concept that connects to another idea or concept, and it usually follows a linear thread. A transition in a story seems to be a natural segue. A natural segue is often fueled by emotion. In the case of tapping, each transition and/or segue is fed by the release of an emotion.

A transition is also an opportunity to move forward. It is also can be the start of a new phase, idea, or concept.

In an EFT tapping script, a transition is a connector between ideas and concepts. It is also an opportunity to move forward, because we have worked through the emotion via tapping. It is an actual change from one state to another.

If you are doing this at home, you watch for the transition to happen. I spent many years doing EFT with humans and their animals over the phone and not being able to see them. I relied heavily on my own intuition.

I did it one of two ways: I either tapped with them and practically had my eyes closed, possibly even pacing, and when I would feel a yawn coming on or a shift in my own body, I knew that the transition was coming and we had relieved the particular emotion we were tapping on. The other way I did it was I often tapped on my own dog, Isabella. Isabella was a healer in her own right and took pride in her job as the surrogate for the animal I was tapping with. As she shifted around, changed her breathing or relaxed even more, I took that as the sign that the animal I was working with remotely was shifting and I would make the transition then.

I share that because we have to start to notice the very subtle shifting in our own being. Obviously, when you are tapping for yourself, you will start to feel the transitions. If you are sitting across the table from a human and are tapping with them, you will see their eyes well up with tears, you will hear their voice fluctuate, and you will notice and understand that things are shifting. But for an animal, it won't always seem so obvious—though I do have a very emotional horse who often lets out a tear when we do EFT tapping sessions around her past.

A Release

A transition in the EFT tapping (script) experience is followed by a *release*. Every now and then, you may feel like the animal or human is resisting the release and you have to use your intuition to transition to another phase of the tapping script. We will talk about that more in Chapter 10.

In a perfect world, we get to experience the release and see the animal release before our very eyes. Sometimes, we have to trust our intuition that this healing technique is working, even if the cat is just staring at you, like, "Can we be done with this, please?"

As far as a release for an animal goes, I will share an excerpt from my book *Energy Healing for Animals,* because I talk extensively in there about how to notice when an animal is soaking-in the healing:

Many of these techniques will mention relaxing the animal into the parasympathetic nervous system. The autonomic nervous system controls most of our bodily functions that we don't have to think about; i.e., heart, digestion, circulation, endocrine, reproduction, etc. The sympathetic nervous system is responsible for our "fight or flight" responses. The parasympathetic nervous system is our "rest and digest" responses as it's the body in a more relaxed state. This is necessary for healing. Remember the inherent intelligence of all bodies: balance.

Aside from feeling good about giving bodywork, or some subtle little touching technique, you will see telltale signs that you are in fact impacting your dog, cat, or horse. You are looking for the signs of relaxation, the signs that the animal has stepped out of fight or flight and into a parasympathetic nervous system, which stimulates relaxation.

Some of the signs you will see are a change in breathing, licking and chewing, yawning, passing gas, and a softness in the eye. When you know an animal has a lot of armor and isn't giving into the healing, taking nice big loud breaths yourself will remind the animal to breathe. Like humans, when finishing with a massage or healing session, the bathroom is the first place the person or animal heads to afterward.

Signs

For dogs, yawning signals to other dogs (or other beings in the multi-species household) that he/she is relaxed. Inherently, a dog knows to yawn to calm itself down. A cat will yawn for the same reasons and also as if to say, "Whatever!" For cats, it is a form of dominance to say, "Hey, I am so chilled!" Cats will also squint at you when they are completely relaxed. At first you might think you are making it up!

A horse will yawn consecutively in a healing or training session to release endorphins. This creates a calming effect on his/her own nervous system.

When a horse does what horse people call licking and chewing, they are releasing some pressure, some tension, or coming down a notch with their level of anxiety. Licking and chewing can indicate processing while training, also.

For dogs and cats, it looks like swallowing and sometimes even a little lick of their lips is followed up by a good yawn. When referring to licking and chewing with a dog, this is not the same type of incessant licking and chewing of a paw as a result of an allergy or anxiousness. This is licking and chewing the air, so to speak.

And as gross as it is, a great sign of knowing you are getting into their system on some level is when they pass gas!

Transitional Phrases

Having a basic understanding as to why an animal might be stuck in a behavior helps with the transitional statements to move through the emotions. Some of these transitional statements are the key to the whole release. Here are some examples:

- A dog that has loyalty to the way their old guardian did things.
- A cat that came from a feral colony of cats and vowed to never trust humans.

- A horse that was hand-fed too much in the past and is now nippy and head shy at the same time.

The language around these transitions can refer back to what is going on for the human and/or the animal. We might not know the animal's past, but we know that they are stuck in a pattern. Some of these phrases will help you come up with a transition statement. You just have to play with it.

Below you'll find some sample transition sentences:

- **Secondary Gain – Human**
  "I realize that if my horse stays lame, I don't have to go to the horse show. I will definitely let this go."

- **Secondary Gain – Animal**
  "If I stay lame, I don't have to go to the show and I get a lot of attention. But I'm missing out on other fun. I'm ready to let this go."

- **Familiarity – Human**
  "This chaos with my animals is so familiar. My household growing up was just this way. But I'm ready to release that now."

- **Familiarity – Animal**
  "This is so fun. It reminds me of my litter mates. We were just CRAZY. But now my person is always mad at me."

- **Blocks – Human**
  "Clearly I'm blocking myself. I'm really good at that. I keep feeling like I can't even potty train a puppy. WTF? OMG, I'm really ready to let that go."

- **Blocks – Animal**
  "I have to pee in the house. I'm afraid to pee out there.
  I don't feel safe. But maybe I can let this go. I am safe outside.
  I am safe."

- **Resistance – Human**
  "Crap, I have such resistance to creating boundaries.
  I know that the cat is affected by it. I'm really ready to put my
  big girl/guy panties on and step up."

- **Resistance – Animal**
  "Maybe I have resistance around peeing in the litter box! I can
  let that go. I can just pee in the litter box. I'm happy to pee in
  the litter box."

- **Battles – Human**
  "All I do is yell at my dog for barking at the neighbor dogs at
  the fence. I feel so mean. I'm sick of being in a constant battle.
  Maybe this is just fun. Maybe I should drop the battle. I'm
  willing to let it go. I hereby drop this stupid battle."

- **Battles – Animal**
  "Those stupid neighbor dogs at the fence, I'll show them. Oh,
  wait, I haven't so far! I could let this battle go"

- **Beliefs – Human**
  "My last animal was so traumatized and never let go of her
  trauma, I can never help this poor little dog."

- **Beliefs – Animal**
  "My last person was so mean, and he always wore a hat. I believe
  all men with hats are mean. Well, maybe not this guy."

- **Vows – Human**
  "Clearly this animal has made some sort of vow to the feral
  community and will never sit in my lap. I'm really ready to let
  go of my need for this cat to be a lap cat. I release my need to
  break her sacred vow."

- **Vows – Animal**
  "My mom was feral, and I made a vow to never trust humans.
  Of course, she would want me to be happy."

- **Loyalties – Human**
  "This new horse is nothing like my last horse. I can't even bond with them. I can't even see them. I miss my old horse. I would really love to be with my old horse. This is not my horse. I am seeing how loyal I am to an animal that no longer exists. I can be loyal to my old horse and see this new horse. I accept and release my loyalties. I am free to feel the loss of the old horse and see who this new horse is."

- **Loyalties – Animal**
  "I have big shoes to fill. She can't even see me. All she thinks about is the other horse/dog/cat. I wish I could be that good. Maybe she will see who I am."
  OR
  "This new person is a jerk. They don't get who I am. It's so much easier to shut down, because they don't see me like my old person did."

Don't Back Away from the Big Feelings

Susie, an equine massage therapist and student of mine, was so sure she had "screwed up a client's horse" with her tapping. She asked in class if that was possible. I didn't answer directly (knowing she couldn't possibly) but asked some key questions.

What I was able to discover is that there was a very angry horse at a barn owned by a young girl. Susie said it was quite obvious that they did not get along.

When I asked her why she thought she had screwed up the tapping for this horse, she replied: "Well, first I promised that now they were going to get along well and everything was going to be glorious from here on out and then after I promised the horse everything, we all found out he had a metabolic issue, got laminitis, and is now lame. The girl is going to let go of the horse. I feel so terrible. I lied to the horse."

I asked her if there were any transitions.

She said: "No, I tried to stay in all the positive emotions."

I reminded her that emotions don't have to be negative or positive, feelings are like ocean waves: They come and go. Some of the bigger feelings are part of our navigational system and are necessary for our growth. Through EFT, we are here to facilitate the release of the bigger feelings.

I also shared that she didn't lie to the horse. Nobody knew the diagnosis at that time, and you could go back and tap again and share with the horse what was going on.

When I tuned into the horse for Susie in class, I felt the horse had a headache. I said to Susie, "If I were this guy walking around with a headache all the time and nobody noticed, and people kept riding me, I'd be pissed, too."

I shared that being mad all the time is going to shake things up for the humans; it gets attention. Unfortunately, he wasn't getting the attention he needed to address the headache.

Susie piped up, "The last two times I massaged him and did a medical intuition scan, he had a headache."

"Yeah, I'd be pissed, too," I said.

Then I reminded her: "The first part of the tapping has to be all of the hard stuff—the angry feelings, the frustrations. EFT tapping truly is telling a hard story while tapping on *feel-good* points, acupressure points that actually calm the system. You should be so in his story with him there should be f-bombs flying. When you feel that releasing or relief from him, then you transition into the perfect world."

Susie processed that for a moment. She realized what had happened and knew that she hadn't screwed him up more; in fact, she is going back to tap on him.

What happens when an animal doesn't shift? You manufacture the transition after several rounds of staying on one emotion. Like people, animals can have lots of wounding and armor. To break through it can be tough.

My own horse, Gabrielle, is very private. She will let students tap on her and will press her lips together and appear not to be fazed by the work, and then she will let it all out by turning her head away from the crowd and yawning so big I can see down her throat. She does this when she thinks no one is looking. I love to use her for that demonstration specifically, to demonstrate what it is like to tap on a stoic animal.

Intuition comes into play when we are finding where to transition when we have a stoic animal. Tapping on the big emotions several rounds (all seven of the points) will have an impact. That's where trust comes into play. You have to trust in your intention and intuition and just go with it, even if your cat is looking at you like, "Stop!"

In the end, the script provides you with a plan of action. Even if you don't use the script itself while tapping, eventually you may just fly by the seat of your pants because you are so good at it.

To create the script, you start with the investigation questions. Below you will find where to get started.

I always feel like the healing begins when someone tells me their story. It is one of the reasons I love animal communication so much. I always say I love energy healing so much I wrote a book about it, but my favorite healing modality will always remain, animal communication.

Why? Because the only requirement is listening. And when someone feels heard, that is healing.

While I'm investigating, hearing the story, I take notes. Maybe the notes are going to end up in the script, and maybe not. But I take a lot of notes.

The Investigation for the Human

I have created a list of questions to get to the heart of the matter. It is based on the handouts from my weekend EFT workshops or the longer courses to train practitioners in my school, CWALU. As noted earlier, in Part Two of this book there are more targeted scripts, but we will get started here.

Below, you will find a blank script to work from. Below that is a script filled out with a fake problem. Who knows, maybe it's real for you!

Investigation for the Human

When my animal does ....

I feel ....

I also feel ....

I continue to feel ....

People around me think ....

....

Which makes me feel even more ....

....

Pick One of the Following:

If I'm honest, I may be getting a secondary gain of ....

....

It's familiar and reminds me of ....

....

Pick One of the Following Transition Setups:

I am feeling blocked/resistant to shift/I'm in a big battle because ....

....

I struggle with my deep-seated belief/vow/loyalty to my feelings because

....

Big Forgiveness or Letting-Go Transition Statement

Pick One of the Following Transition Setups:

- I forgive myself. I am ready to let this go.
- It's time to move on.
- I'm ready to try something new.
- I can't take it anymore.

In a perfect world my animal companion would ....

....

And we would feel ....

....

NOTE: I would say to pick only one transition setup and one transition statement. Sometimes, though, more than one may apply, because there are so many complex issues involved from the past and present. If that is the case, you could do one of two things:

1. Use only both of the transition statements to tap on, or
2. Make a note of the other big emotion/complexity/situation involved, and tap on it in a separate second or third round of tapping.

Below you will find the script filled out with a fake problem. Let's pretend that a person adopts a dog after the loss of her other dog, Donny. This new dog drives her crazy because he barks too much. Let's break it down. I have written this out in such a way that you can see the question in the investigation, such as "When my animal does .... ," and beneath it, an example *answer*.

The Issue

When my animal does ....

When my dog, Buddy, barks incessantly,

I feel ....

I feel like a knife is going through my forehead.

I also feel ....

I feel like I can't concentrate. ....

The Experience

I continue to feel ....

I feel frustrated.
I am so frustrated.
Nothing works.
I feel mad.
I feel mad.
I feel like I can't control my dog.
I feel like my dog doesn't give a crap about how I feel.

People around me think ....

People around me think I can't control my silly dog.

Which makes me feel even more ....

Which makes me feel incompetent as a pet parent.

The Middle Transition (try to pick one):

If I'm honest, I may be getting a secondary gain of ....

....

> *I don't have to get that close to Buddy, because I'm always so mad at him.*

It's familiar and reminds me of ....

....

> *He's so not like Donny.*
> *Donny was perfect.*
> *Buddy makes me crazy.*
> *I feel terrible for even saying that.*
> *I am a bad dog person.*
> *I can't control my dog.*
> *It makes me sad, because I don't love him like I could.*

The Transition Setup (try to pick one):

I am feeling blocked/resistant to shift/I'm in a big battle,

because ....

....

I struggle with my deep-seated belief/vow/loyalty to my feelings,

because ....

> *I have such deep loyalty to the other dog, Donny, who passed on two years ago. If I'm totally honest with myself, I am always mad at my dog, Buddy.*
> *I didn't realize how much my grief over Donny is controlling me.*
> *So much grief.*
> *I still miss Donny.*
> *He was perfect.*
> *I didn't realize how much grief I have.*

I am still grieving.

I have so much grief.

I am grieving.

Transition Statement (try to pick one):

- ☐ I forgive myself. I am ready to let this go (statement can be reversed).
- ☐ It's time to move on.
- ☐ I'm ready to try something new.
- ☐ I can't take it anymore.

....

I am really ready to let this go. I forgive myself.

And I forgive Buddy. Buddy is just being Buddy.

The Outcome

In a perfect world our animal companion and I would ....

....

In a perfect world, I have forgiven myself.

And we would feel ....

....

And Buddy and I are closer for it.

I have tapped into the deep grief with Donny and am letting him go even more.

I am fully accepting Buddy.

I am seeing Buddy for who he is.

I love Buddy.

And because I've discovered this, we feel even more connected to each other.

We only have fun and respect for each other.

We listen to each other.

And we feel more in love than ever.

The Investigation for the Animal

Now, you may be an animal communicator and can find out all of the details that motivate the dog to bark or whatever your challenge is. If you haven't already developed your animal communication muscle, as the guardian, you may find it difficult to get neutral enough to be able to find out what is the underlying struggle that makes the dog *seem* obstinate, because, to you, it just seems like they are being obstinate.

In order to create a neutral script, if you aren't skilled at animal communication, you could try one of four things:

1. Hire an animal communicator to help you understand from the animal's worldview.
2. You could wing it, and answer the questions in the investigation to the best of your ability!
3. You could do the little meditation in the sidebar.
4. You could do a "what if" exercise. Take a blank piece of paper, and almost as if you are automatic writing, find out what is motivating your beloved. See below in the second sidebar. NOTE: The meditation and the automatic writing exercises are actually great to do together.

MEDITATION: *Getting Neutral*

Take a few minutes to just breathe into the bottom of your feet. With each breath, imagine you are letting go of any physical, mental and emotional bits and pieces that stand in the way of you getting to a neutral space. Imagine that you are completely neutral.

MEDITATION: *What If?*

Take a moment to center. Feel your feet solidly on the ground. Close your eyes and feel into your animal companion. Now, write down whatever comes to mind with the following questions:

- What if I'm this dog/cat/horse/bird/ferret/other, and I love to .... ?
- How am I feeling about this?
- What are the sensations?
- Does it invigorate me?
- Does it intimidate me?
- What are the other feelings involved with this?

Here is the script you will be working from. Again, these are handouts from my workshops. It's a great jumping-off point. We will look at the blank script first and then we will look at it from the point of view of Buddy, the barking dog.

Investigation for the Animal

When I ....

OR

When .... happens,

I feel ....

I also feel ....

I continue to feel ....

People around me think ....

....

Which makes me feel even more ....

....

Pick One of the Following:

If I'm honest, I may be getting a secondary gain of ....

....

It's familiar and reminds me of ....

....

Pick One of the Following Transition Setups:

I am feeling blocked/resistant to shift/I'm in a big battle, because ....

....

I struggle with my deep-seated belief/vow/loyalty to my feelings,

because ....

Big Forgiveness or Letting-Go Transition Statement

Pick One of the Following Transition Setups:

- [ ] I forgive myself. I am ready to let this go (statement can be reversed).
- [ ] It's time to move on.
- [ ] I'm ready to try something new.
- [ ] I can't take it anymore.

In a perfect world my person and I would ....

....

And we would feel ....

....

Let's look at our Buddy-the-barking-dog scenario and the human that hates the barking and break this down into the sequence. Now we get to be Buddy and share his perspective on the issue in question. Buddy's views are stated in italics beneath the statement prompts.

The Issue

When I ....

When I bark, I am alerting the world that I am alive.

OR

When .... happens,

When I bark, I am alerting the world that I am alive.

I feel ....

alive!

I also feel ....

responsible

The Experience

I continue to feel ....

*I need to let everyone know what is going on! I am letting my
    person/people know.*
I am letting the neighborhood know.
You can't believe what walks by the house!
Wow!

People around me think ....

People around me think I'm annoying.
I feel sad.
My person is always on the computer.
I'm not trying to be annoying.
I'm trying to be helpful.
Nobody sees it.

Which makes me feel even more ....

....

I'm afraid they are missing out!
*Which makes me feel even more committed to letting them know
    of the dangers.*
I'm afraid they don't know what is going on!
I actually get afraid for them!
I'm afraid!
I'm afraid!
*I'm afraid that nobody will help me if one of those giant dogs out
    there came into the yard.*
I just don't feel safe with these dogs around.
I'm afraid that nobody's got my back.
I will have to bark louder.
I have to bark louder.
Nobody seems to notice me.
I am trying to save our lives, for crying out loud!

Let's say you pick:

It's familiar and reminds me of ....

> *This is so familiar.*
> *In my first home, I was trying to save the world.*
> *Nobody noticed.*
> *They were always mad at me.*
> *The neighbors were mad.*
> *This is so familiar.*

The Transition Setup (try to pick one):

I am feeling blocked/resistant to shift/I'm in a big battle, because ....

....

I struggle with my deep-seated belief/vow/loyalty to my feelings,

because ....

Let's say you pick:

I am feeling blocked/resistant to shift/I'm in a big battle, because ....

....

> *It's familiar.*

The Transition Statement (try to pick one):

- [ ] I forgive myself. I am ready to let this go (statement can be reversed).
- [ ] It's time to move on.
- [ ] I'm ready to try something new.
- [ ] I can't take it anymore.
- [ ] I'm ready to try something new.

....

> *I am so ready to try something new.*
> *I don't even know what that would be.*
> *My person doesn't seem to give a crap about what is walking by.*

In fact, he/she/they shut(s) the door.
And then I feel really lonely.
I am so lonely.
I am ready to try something new.
I am trying something new.
I may have to just lie in his/her/their office at his/her/their feet.
I am trying something new now.

The Outcome

In a perfect world ....

In a perfect world, I am confident.

And we would feel ....

We would feel so great together.
I am confident.
I am confident.
I am confident.
I am strong.
I would rather be cozy in his/her/their office.
I would rather be close to him/her/them.
We would feel cozy when he/she/they are working.
We would face adventure together.
I would trust him/her/them.
He/she/they would trust me.
Oh, I love this world!
This world is yummy and safe.
We are all safe together.
Together we are safe.

On the one hand, creating a script for tapping can seem complex; on the other, tapping is simple, affective, *and* effective—especially, once you get the hang of it. To be honest, the healing begins the minute pen hits the paper; that is, creating notes to tap on is already starting the process on a profound level. As I have mentioned above, healing starts with listening. EFT tapping is an opportunity for all parties to listen to each other.

Still to come in Chapter 4 is the "setup statement," which involves tapping on a specific point while making an overview statement, or "setting up" what is to come, even previewing the desired outcome to some degree. I left it out in this chapter as I didn't want to complicate the investigation and the work needed to create the script (the vegan sandwich meat, if you will).

While developing a script may seem daunting, remember: This is not "Great Script Freedom Technique" nor is it "Intellectual Freedom Technique"; it is Emotional Freedom Technique. As long as you can identify key feelings and emotions running in the background for you and your animal, this should help your script along. If your script only identifies key emotions and taps on those emotions without a big story, without a big script, you are still going to see some shifts.

The next step is actually tapping.

4

Let's Tap

By now you should be well acquainted with the simple premise of Emotional Freedom Technique, aka EFT or tapping: By lightly tapping on feel-good acupressure points, you can unlock emotional baggage, triggers, belief systems, and/or traumatic stories and release them from your system. You have learned why it's important to have this tool in your tool box when your animals need healing at any level of their being, and you know how to create the script that goes along with the tapping.

Now it's time to get into the nuts and bolts of tapping. Where do you tap? How do you tap?

Full details ahead, but for a quick overview, you can tap on specified points on one side of the body or both sides, using two fingers or more. While there are many acupressure points along the 14 meridians of Traditional Chinese Medicine, each tapping point that has been selected for this energetic technique has a strong and specific purpose, and we'll get into all of that in this chapter.

Let's begin by building on the last chapter and learn how to create the "setup statement."

The Setup Statement

When tapping on humans, start by establishing a setup statement, a description of the situation you are addressing. You will repeat this statement as you tap along the center point of the outside edge of your hand. This is also known as the "karate chop point." A setup statement not only sets up the story but starts to convey the emotions involved.

Often, you will choose three setup statements and then end with phrases like "And I love and accept myself" or "I honor the choices I'm making." I use both of these frequently, and interchangeably. Sometimes, you can tell the whole story of an event that caused deeply held emotions to start swirling under the surface and then move into the tapping points on the face and chest while reviewing those emotions.

Starting simply with the setup statement allows for those bigger emotions to well up to be released. If I were tapping on the human who had to handle Shakespeare in Chapter 1, I might try these:

- Even though my horse is a total bully and is scaring the *crap* out of me, I love and accept myself.
- Even though my horse is acting like a total nut job—I don't even know this guy right now—and I'm not even sure what to do, I love and accept myself.
- Even though I really don't know what to do and I hate seeing these kids so terrified on their ponies, I honor the choices I'm making by staying here and working it out.

Tapping Sequences

Let's review the physical locations of the tapping points on the body first. Later, we will break down what they're used for according to Traditional Chinese Medicine. We'll start with tapping for people, for reasons we've covered in earlier chapters: Animals follow our lead, which can create a vicious cycle of difficult emotions if the human aspect is not addressed. Also, the human usually carries the bigger emotional charge around an event, so it's good to start by releasing that. Once we have worked through the layers of the human's emotional response—fear, for instance—it's easier for the animal to release its own fear through tapping on their behalf.

The Tapping Sequence for Humans

Start by tapping on the setup/karate chop point, the center point on the outside edge of the hand, then tap on:

1. Inside the eye socket – on the bone, where the eyebrow starts.
2. Outside the eye socket – on the bone, about 1/8th inch under the outside of the brow.
3. Under the eye – on the bone, directly under the center of the eye.
4. Under the nose – on the fleshy part between nose and upper lip.
5. Under the lips – on the crease between the lower lip and the chin.
6. Collarbone – just below the collarbone, in the center, at the little indentation.
7. Top of the head – just that, on the crown of the head.

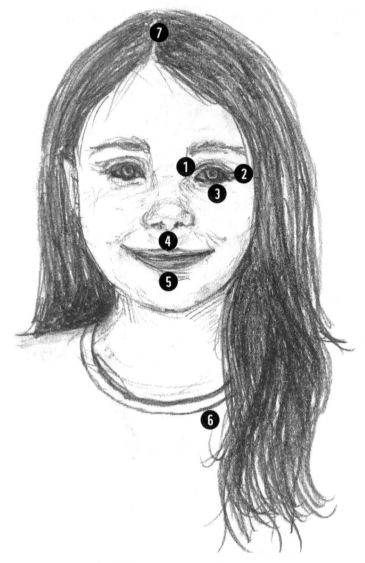

The Tapping Points on a Human

Once you get familiar with tapping, as long as you're working with a person, you can also add the point under the armpit. I have taken it out of my tapping world, because when I'm tapping on animals and I'm working on an aggressive dog, an antsy horse, or a persnickety cat, reaching around to the side can create a reaction. It was easier for the safety of all to omit that point, and it is not essential to keep it in the human sequence either, so I decided to drop it altogether.

The Tapping Sequence for Dogs and Cats

When it comes to tapping on dogs and cats, the traditional setup statement/karate chop point on a dog or a cat would be down by their front ankle. It is such an awkward place for an animal, and I discovered that it is often a reactive point for them, too, so again, I have left that point out.

That said, you can do the karate chop point on yourself for the animal's setup statement. Since I usually do tapping for the human before I work on the animal, the situation has already been "set up," or framed, and it is a matter of taking that framing from the human to tapping on the animal. Also, if you happen to be an animal communicator yourself, you can do a session with the animal before tapping on them. Then you will hear the animal's version of whatever upsetting event may have happened, and you can get the setup or framing established that way.

Once you've used one of these methods to get the setup nailed down, use this sequence:

1. Inside the eye socket – on the bone, right next to the inside of the eye socket.
2. Outside the eye socket – on the bone, right next to the outside of the eye socket.
3. Under the eye – on the bone, directly under the center of the eye.
4. On the nose – technically, this acupressure point would be on the upper lip between the nostrils; as a precaution against nipping or biting, you might place your *intention* on that point and then tap on the top of the nose where the wet snout (the rhinarium) and the fur come together.
5. Chin – where the lips and the fur meet on the lower jaw.
6. Chest – on either side of the breastbone (sternum), between the breastbone and the shoulder (scapula), where there is a little indentation.
7. Top of the head – just that, on the crown of the head.

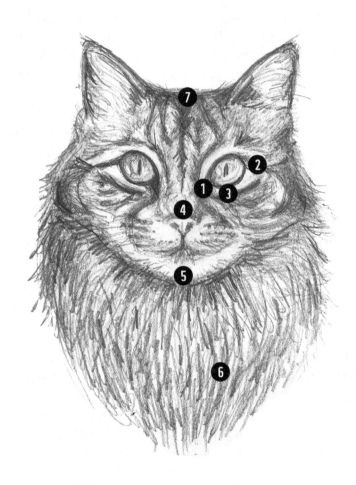

The Tapping Points on a Cat

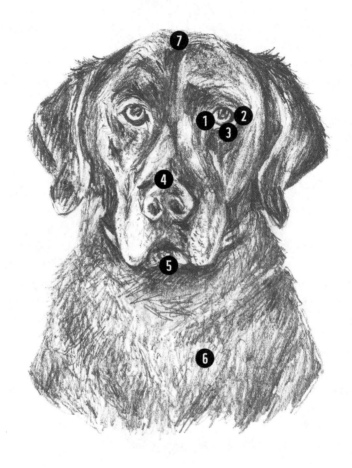

The Tapping Points on a Dog

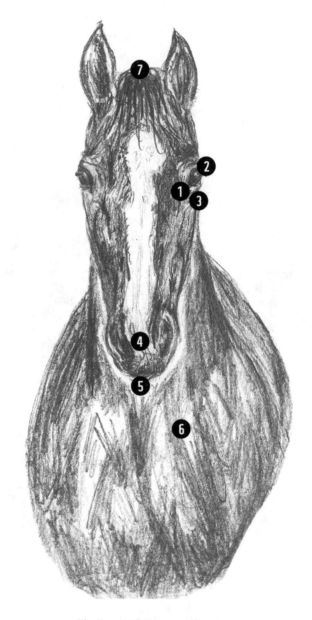

The Tapping Points on a Horse

The Tapping Sequence for Horses

When it comes to tapping on horses, the setup statement/karate chop point happens to be right above the ankle bone (called the fetlock on a horse) on the front legs, and it would be awkward to start by bending down to tap there and then work on their faces. We want to be mindful of their state of being when we are tapping on them, and if you know horses, you always want to err on the side of caution.

Therefore, as I did for dogs and cats, I have left the setup statement out of this sequence. You can also use the workarounds I discovered for creating a setup statement described in the Dogs and Cats section above.

From there, it's:

1. Inside the eye socket – the bone next to the inside of the eye socket.
2. Outside the eye socket – on the bone, next to the outside of the eye socket.
3. Under the eye—on the bone, directly under the center of the eye.
4. On the nose – technically, this acupressure point is on the upper lip between the nostrils, but it is best to air-tap as a precaution against nipping or biting.
5. Chin – under the lower lip.
6. Chest – on either side of the breastbone (sternum), between the breastbone and the shoulder (scapula), where there is a little indentation.
7. Top of the head – just that, on the crown of the head.

What the Specific Points Are Used For

If you're like me when I'm lying on an acupuncture table and the doctor is carefully and strategically placing various needles in my body, you'll want to know what it all means. Why does stimulating a given point cause the sensation I experience? Some points are painful, while others make me want to pass out from sheer bliss. I have a million questions when the acupuncturist is working on the painful points, and then, eventually, according to the strategic plan, the doctor hits the bliss points, and I'm out. I've learned a lot about tapping from being on the acupuncture table.

I fell in love with the power of acupressure when I started working on one of my own horses. Later, acupressure became a very important component of my practice as an animal communicator. While I didn't continue doing it as a professional practitioner of acupressure, per se, I still use the method every day. And now I have joined with Dr. Jill Todd, holistic veterinarian, to offer acupressure classes through my school. This has renewed my love affair with acupressure and allowed me to dive deeper into this ancient technology and healing method, a deeper dive that I can now share with you.

Now, if you simply want to get tapping and couldn't care less about what it all means, you can skip this section. But if you are interested in learning the theory beneath it all, read on. It can definitely be helpful to have this background. For example, certain points can offer more potent healing for your animal than other points, or be more calming. If you know this ahead of time, you can hone right in on the points that are likely to work best for your situation.

Physical and Emotional Indications for the Points in Traditional Chinese Medicine

Indications in Humans

What Does the Karate Chop Point Do?

On the human chart, we start with the Karate Chop (KC) point, Small Intestine (SI) 3, for the setup statement. (There's more on setup statements and what to say below.) Because the sister meridian for the Small Intestine is the Heart meridian, the SI meridian is associated with protecting the heart, as well as taking in and absorbing nutrients, physically, emotionally, and spiritually.

Physically, this point literally alleviates neck pain and stress in the neck—both places where we hold tension. It also alleviates stress in our gut and small intestine. It is known to balance the heart and mind, releasing what is heavy in the heart and thereby opening the mind.

What follows is a summary of the functions of each of the points you will be tapping. For each, I have listed the names and numbers of the points (which are named according to their placement along a meridian); alternate names for the specific meridians, to give you another way to think about them; the related element, where applicable; physical indications for using that point; and emotional indications for using the point.

I have also repeated the locations of the points, as when I teach tapping to beginners, I say them aloud. After you've been tapping for a while, you will no longer need these cues.

1. **Bladder 1 (BL 1):** inside of the eye socket – on the bone, right where the eyebrow starts
   Bladder Meridian: the Great Mediator
   Element: water
   Physical Indications: good for eye disorders, eye discharge, dry eye, nasal disorders, sinus disorders, challenges with the nervous system
   Emotional Indications: very calming

2. **Triple Heater 23 (TH 23):** outside of the eye socket – on the bone, about 1/8th inch under the outside of the brow
   Triple Heater Meridian: the Commander of All Energies (this does not correspond to an organ but to a series of organs, or a system)
   Element: fire
   Physical Indications: great for trigeminal and facial nerve issues, vertigo, head pain, epilepsy, and dry eye; relieves pain
   Emotional Indications: when balanced, brings joy, kindheartedness

3. **Stomach 1 (ST 1):** under the eye – up by the lower lid, about 1/8th inch under and in line with the pupil
   Stomach Meridian: the Sea of Nourishment
   Element: earth
   Physical Indications: anything involving the face, teeth, jaws, or eyes; facial paralysis
   Emotional Indications: worry, anxiety, nervousness; when balanced, calm and collected

Stomach 2 (ST 2): under the eye between the lower lid and the bone, in line with the pupil
Stomach Meridian: the Sea of Nourishment
Element: earth
Physical Indications: eye issues, sinus congestion, clarity of vision; clears heat; relaxes tendons and ligaments

Because these two points are close together, you are often hitting both points when you tap on this area.

4. **Governing Vessel 26 (GV 26):** under the nose – on the fleshy part between the nose and the upper lip
   Governing Vessel Meridian: the Sea of Yang, governing all yang energies
   Physical Indications: an emergency point for shock, collapse, heatstroke, seizures, respiratory stimulation, and trauma; referred to as the "first aid point"
   Emotional Indications: one of the best calming points on the body

5. **Conception Vessel 24 (CV 24):** under the lips – on the crease between the lower lip and the chin
   Conception Vessel Meridian: the Sea of Yin, governing all yin energies
   Physical Indications: helps mouth issues, gingivitis, and tooth pain
   Emotional Indications: relieves fear and anxiety

6. **Kidney 27 (KI 27):** collarbone – just below the collarbone in the center, where there is a little indentation
   Kidney Meridian: Residence of Resolution
   Element: water
   Physical Indications: cough, asthma, respiratory conditions; strengthens immune system
   Emotional Indications: relieves anxiety and mental tiredness

Alternatively you could tap on LU 1 to relieve deep grief. And you could tap with all four fingers and reach both KI 27 and LU 1 for the ultimate relief from deeply sad or traumatic events.

Lung 1 (LU 1): collarbone – just under the clavicle toward the shoulder
Lung Meridian: Controller of Receiving Chi
Element: metal
Physical Indications: cough, wheezing, asthma, fullness in chest, shoulder pain, back pain, pain in chest
Emotional Indications: relief of fatigue, grief, and trauma

7. **Governing Vessel 20 (GV 20):** top of the head – just that, on the crown of the head
   Governing Vessel Meridian: This point is considered to be the One Hundred Meeting Points, and this is so true. (There are also many other acupressure points right there on the top of the head, one of which I'll list next.)
   Physical Indications: headache, eye strain, brain dysfunctions
   Emotional Indications: relieves depression and overthinking; brings about clarity of thought and mind

You will also be accessing:

Bladder Meridian 6 (BL 6): top of the head, but just off the center line
Bladder Meridian: Guardian of Peace
Element: water
Physical indications: blurry vision, dizziness
Emotional indications: relieves frustration, vexation

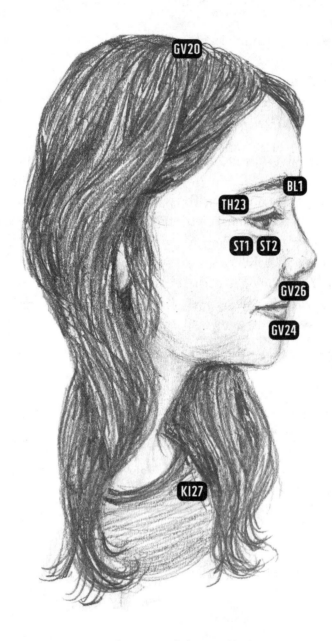

Acupressure Points on a Human

Indications in Dogs and Cats

1. **Bladder 1 (BL 1):** inside of the eye socket – on the bone, right next to the inside of the eye
   Bladder Meridian: Guardian of Peace
   Element: water
   Physical Indications: good for eye disorders, eye discharge, dry eye, nasal disorders, sinus disorders, challenges with the nervous system
   Emotional Indications: very calming

2. **Triple Heater 23 (TH 23):** outside of the eye socket – on the bone, right next to the outside of the eye
   Triple Heater Meridian: the Commander of All Energies (this does not correspond to an organ but to a series of organs, or a system)
   Element: fire
   Physical indications: trigeminal and facial nerve issues, vertigo, head pain, epilepsy, and dry eye; relieves pain
   Emotional indications: when balanced, brings joy, kindheartedness

3. **Stomach 1 (ST 1):** under the eye – on the bone in line with the pupil
   Stomach Meridian: the Sea of Nourishment
   Element: earth
   Physical Indications: anything involving the face, teeth, jaws, eyes; facial paralysis
   Emotional Indications: worry, anxiety, nervousness; when balanced, calm and collected

   Stomach 2 (ST 2): under the eye between the lower lid and the bone, in line with the pupil
   Stomach Meridian: the Sea of Nourishment
   Element: earth
   Physical indications: eye issues, sinus congestion, clarity of vision; clears heat; relaxes tendons and ligaments

   Because these two points are close together, you are often hitting both points when you tap on this area.

4. **Governing Vessel 26 (GV 26):** on the nose – technically, this acupressure point would be on the upper lip between the nostrils; as a precaution against nipping or biting, you might place your "intention" on that point and then tap on the top of the nose where the wet snout (the rhinarium) and the fur come together

    Physical Indications: emergency point for shock, collapse, heatstroke, seizures, respiratory stimulation, and trauma; referred to as the "first aid point"

    Emotional Indications: one of the best calming points on the body

5. **Conception Vessel 24 (CV 24):** under the lips – the crease between the lower lip and the chin

    Conception Vessel Meridian: the Sea of Yin, governing all yin energies

    Physical Indications: helps mouth issues, gingivitis, and tooth pain

    Emotional Indications: relieves fear and anxiety

6. **Kidney 27 (KI 27):** collarbone – on either side of the breastbone, between the breastbone (sternum) and the shoulder (scapula), where there is a little indentation

    Kidney Meridian: Residence of Resolution

    Element: water

    Physical Indications: cough, asthma, respiratory conditions; strengthens immune system

    Emotional Indications: relieves anxiety and mental tiredness

Alternatively you could tap on Lung 1 to relieve deep grief. And you could tap with all four fingers and reach both KI 27 and LU 1 for the ultimate relief from deeply sad or traumatic events.

Lung 1 (LU 1): collarbone, in the hollow of the chest, just under the foreleg, toward the shoulder

Lung Meridian: Controller of Receiving Chi

Element: metal

Physical Indications: cough, wheezing, asthma, fullness in chest, shoulder pain, back pain, pain in chest

Emotional Indications: relief for fatigue, grief, and trauma

7. **Governing Vessel 20 (GV 20):** top of the head – just that, the crown of the head

   Governing Vessel Meridian: This point is considered to be the One Hundred Meeting Points, and this is so true. (There are also many other acupressure points right there on the top of the head, one of which I'll list next.)

   Physical Indications: headache, eye strain, brain dysfunctions

   Emotional Indications: relieves depression and overthinking; brings about clarity of thought and mind

You will also be accessing:

Bladder Meridian 6 (BL 6): top of the head, but just off the center line

Bladder Meridian: Guardian of Peace

Element: water

Physical Indications: blurry vision, dizziness

Emotional Indications: relieves frustration, vexation

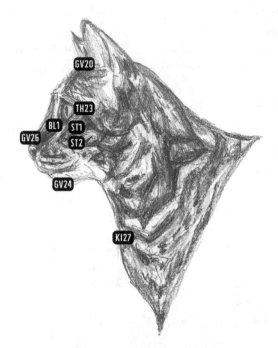

Acupressure Points on a Cat

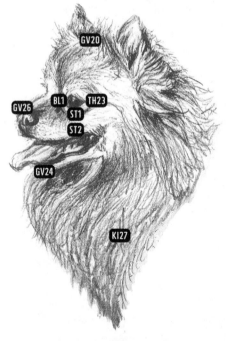

Acupressure Points on a Dog

Indications in Horses

1. **Bladder 1 (BL 1):** inside of the eye socket – the bone right next to the inside of the eye
   Bladder Meridian: Guardian of Peace
   Element: water
   Physical Indications: good for eye disorders, eye discharge, dry eye, nasal disorders, sinus disorders, challenges with the nervous system
   Emotional Indications: very calming

2. **Triple Heater 23 (TH 23):** outside of the eye socket – on the bone, right next to the outside of the eye
   Triple Heater Meridian: the Commander of all Energies (this does not correspond to an organ but to a series of organs, or a system)
   Element: fire
   Physical Indications: trigeminal and facial nerve issues, vertigo, head pain, epilepsy, and dry eye; relieves pain
   Emotional Indications: when balanced, brings joy, kindheartedness

3. **Stomach 1 (ST 1):** under the eye – on the bone, directly in line with the pupil
   Stomach Meridian: the Sea of Nourishment
   Element: earth
   Physical Indications: anything involving the face, teeth, jaws, eyes; facial paralysis
   Emotional Indications: worry, anxiety, nervousness; when balanced, calm and collected

4. **Governing Vessel 26 (GV 26):** on the nose – technically, this acupressure point would be on the upper lip between the nostrils; as a precaution against nipping or biting, you might place your "intention" on that point and tap on the top of the nose where the wet snout (the rhinarium) and the fur come together
   Governing Vessel: the Sea of Yang, governing all yang energies
   Physical Indications: emergency point for shock, collapse, heatstroke, seizures, respiratory stimulation, and trauma; referred to as the "first aid point"
   Emotional Indications: one of the best calming points on the body

5. **Conception Vessel 24 (CV 24):** under the lips

   Conception Vessel Meridian: the Sea of Yin, governing all yin energies

   Physical Indications: helps mouth issues, gingivitis, and tooth pain

   Emotional Indications: relieves fear and anxiety

6. **Kidney 27 (KI 27):** collarbone—on either side of the breastbone (sternum), between the breastbone and the shoulder (scapula), where there is a little indentation

   Kidney Meridian: Residence of Resolution

   Element: water

   Physical Indications: cough, asthma, respiratory conditions, strengthens immune system

   Emotional Indications: relieves anxiety and mental tiredness

   Alternatively you could tap on Lung 1 to relieve deep grief. And you could tap with all four fingers and reach both KI 27 and LU 1 for the ultimate relief from deeply sad or traumatic events.

   Lung 1 (LU 1): collarbone, is in the hollow of the chest, just under the foreleg, toward the shoulder

   Lung Meridian: Controller of Receiving Chi

   Element: metal

   Physical Indications: cough, wheezing, asthma, fullness in chest, shoulder pain, back pain, pain in chest

   Emotional Indications: relief for fatigue, grief and trauma

7. **Governing Vessel 20 (GV 20):** top of the head (in horses, the very top of the head is called the poll)

   Governing Vessel Meridian: the Sea of Yang, governing all yang energies

   This point on the Governing Vessel Meridian is considered to be the One Hundred Meeting Points, and this is so true. (There are also many other acupressure points right there on the top of the head, one of which I'll list next.)

Element: fire

Physical Indications: headache, eye strain, brain dysfunctions

Emotional Indications: relieves depression and overthinking; brings about clarity of thought and mind

You will also be accessing:

Bladder Meridian 10 (BL 10): top of the head but a little behind the poll, toward the shoulder

Bladder Meridian: Guardian of Peace

Element: water

Physical indications: neck, back, and shoulder pain

Emotional indications: relieves anxiety and nervous tension

Gall Bladder 20 (GB 20): also the top of the head, a little behind the poll

Gall Bladder Meridian: the Official of Decision and Judgment

Element: wood

Physical Indications: head and neck tension, eye issues, nasal congestion, and vertigo

Emotional Indications: repressed anger, indecisiveness; when balanced, the passion for life returns

PLEASE NOTE: Horses do not have a gall bladder. This meridian still holds value energetically for the horse, however, because it is mentally, physically, and emotionally a meridian/organ system that process nutrients and emotions in order to move forward in life.

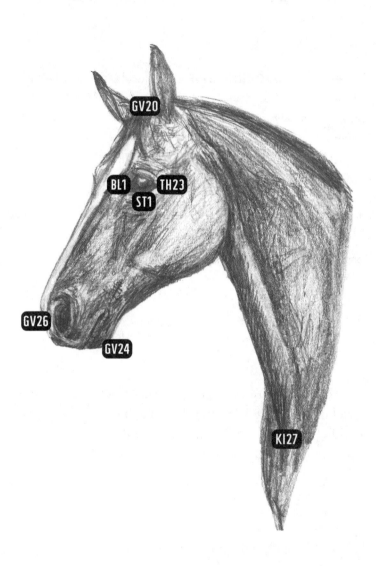

Acupressure Points on a Horse

Alternatives to "Regular" Tapping

EFT Tapping can accelerate as we go along and begin to feel a little more vigorous when we get to particular points that surface and release more emotional energy. We want to be mindful of the animal's degree of sensitivity as we move through the sequence and not necessarily do it "by the book" each time.

Many behavioral issues can have their origins in injuries and aches and pains, so as we're tapping we could accidentally unlock old muscle memory, as well as trigger the emotion that is bound up in it. We always want to be as delicate and mindful as possible.

I teach tapping day in and day out in my school, as well as at workshops elsewhere, so I am prepared for the questions most people ask. Following are the common categories, and I will dive into each one after you read the list:

- Are there other ways to tap?
- What if I can't tap on the animal's face?
- What if I can't tap on them at all?
- What about remote tapping?
- When should I not tap on an animal?

Other Ways to Tap

Right now you are probably thinking, *Okay, Joan, that was amazing information, but what does the gallbladder meridian have to do with my dog and his biting problem? Or this cat's asthma? Or my horse's fear of men wearing hats?*

There are three ways you can tap on, or for, an animal with regard to a behavioral or health challenge:

1. You can tap right on the points I've outlined above, with the indications listed as your guide.
2. Humans can tap on themselves on behalf of their animal, acting as a surrogate.
3. You can tap without actually touching the animal—call it "air tapping."
4. You can tap on another animal as the surrogate.
5. You can tap on a stuffed animal as the surrogate.

If we choose option no. 2 (tapping on ourselves, acting as a surrogate on behalf of our animal companion), as it sounds, we tap on the tapping points on ourselves *while speaking on behalf of the animal.*

What If I Can't Tap on the Animal's Face?

Here are several suggestions. I like to tap on the association points (see the next section), especially when it comes to cats, who can quickly become annoyed and swat at you (claws first) or think you're playing. The association points run along the Bladder Meridian.

Tapping on the Bladder Meridian

The Bladder Meridian has association points connected to each of the organs and all the other meridians. If you work on points along this meridian, you can easily accomplish the same calming or stimulation effects without touching the face. We call these "stand-in" points, *association points.*

Association points can be found all along the Bladder Meridian. The Bladder Meridian goes from the inside of the eye socket (our first tapping point), over the head, and then descends parallel to the spine to the human baby toe, the outside toe on the hind leg of a dog or cat, or the hoof on the hind leg of a horse. When tapping, you would follow the association points from close to the neck down the spine towards the tail. The points correspond to the following organs:

Bladder Meridian Point	Organ
Bl 13	Lung
Bl 14	Pericardium
Bl 15	Heart
Bl 18	Liver
Bl 19	Gall Bladder
Bl 20	Spleen
Bl 21	Stomach
Bl 22	Triple Heater
Bl 23	Kidney
Bl 25	Large Intestine
Bl 27	Small Intestine
Bl 28	Bladder

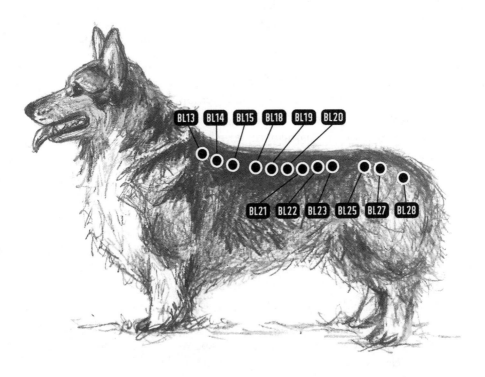

The association points are along the bladder meridian. Each of these points are found on both sides of the spine.

As you are working, association points along the Bladder Meridian can inform you if something is going on with the animal physically. If you find an overly sensitive spot, you might want to look further into which organ is connected to that area. Tapping along this meridian is also very calming to the resistant animal or the animal with deep trauma stored in their body.

What If I Can't Tap on Them at All?

When I first learned tapping, I had already heard about surrogate tapping; that is, tapping on someone or something else on behalf of the one who is in need of support. You can get creative with what you select as a surrogate. You could tap on a stuffed animal or a chart of the acupressure points, or tap on yourself or another animal in your household, while holding the intention for the animal in need. Air tapping is something I do regularly if I can't touch the animal. For example, if I'm in a shelter with an animal that is highly aggressive, I will tap in the air as if I'm accessing each point on their body. Sure, it looks a little weird, but trust me: the intention behind that air tapping brings results.

What about Remote Tapping?

You can extend surrogate tapping and air tapping to working with an animal over the phone or by video, too. I do this all the time in my practice. I might tap on one of my own animals or do some air tapping in solidarity with the client and their animal. I call out the points for the person as I go along, so they know exactly where to go if they're tapping on their own animal as we work through the emotions.

How do you know it's working? The animal tells you. It will release and sigh at all the right places, just as it would if you were tapping on them by touch. (I will review the signs of release on pages 52 and 95.)

When Should I Not Tap on an Animal?

When an animal has been traumatized by human touch, tapping on them might bring on more trauma. This is especially true if they've had any type of head injury at the hands of humans. For this reason, I always steer clear of physically tapping on traumatized, timid, or aggressive animals.

Ultimately, you need to use your intuition to address this question. When you feel into your intuition, do you see the animal relaxing into their story when you tap on these points, or do you sense that they will become more rigid? You do not want rigidity; this is about healing!

At times when I have felt like I shouldn't or couldn't touch a client's animal, and that client has a second dog, cat, or horse, I have done surrogate tapping on the other animal. If the person feels safe tapping on the animal we are healing, they can mirror what I'm doing, and that often works well.

The Value of Touch

Anytime we can touch an animal, especially when we do it with intention, it's a bonus for them. As we reviewed in Chapter 1, animals have the ability to release their story or their emotions through exercise, through movement. For some animals, though, that's not enough—their trauma is too great, or there has been no natural means of expression to release a story, to get to those deep emotions that are stored in the muscle memory in their body.

I just want to underscore this point as you digest the information on points and sequences in this chapter. Bodywork modalities and energetic techniques that involve touch offer the quickest means of helping an animal release their emotional pain.

Signs an Animal Is Releasing: A Review

As we discussed in Chapter 3, animals exhibit release pretty openly, though on occasion you may come across that one very stoic animal. When I approach my own horse Gabrielle to start tapping, she will press her lips together as if to say "You can't help me!" But after the tapping, she can't help but let out a big sigh.

Don't be discouraged if you don't see the telltale signs that an animal is releasing right away, or even see them at all. The animal may be slow to process, or may just be the private type, just as people are at times.

To review, some of the signs to look for are:

1. A change in breathing
2. Licking and chewing
3. Yawning
4. Passing gas
5. A softness in the eye

When you know an animal has a lot of armor and isn't giving in to the healing, like Gabrielle, take some nice, big, loud breaths yourself. This will remind the animal to breathe.

Putting It All Together

Now let's combine the sample tapping script you learned in Chapter 3 with the information about the points and the sequence in this chapter. Here we go!

For the Human

Setup Statement (spoken while tapping on the karate chop point):

- *Even though my dog Buddy barks incessantly, and it drives me insane, I love and accept myself.*
- *Even though my dog Buddy loses his mind when he sees someone walk by the house, and I have to yell at him, I love and accept myself.*
- *Even though my dog Buddy is a bad dog—and I know, there are no bad dogs—maybe it's all my fault, and I honor the choices I've made.*

Tapping through the Points

Inside the eye socket – *When my dog Buddy barks incessantly . . .*
Outside the eye socket – *I feel like a knife is going through my forehead.*
Under the eye – *I can't concentrate.*
Under the nose – *I feel frustrated.*
Under the bottom lip – *I feel mad.*
Collarbone – *I feel like I can't control my dog.*
Top of the head – *I feel like my dog doesn't give a crap about how I feel.*
Inside the eye socket – *People around me think I can't control my dang dog . . .*
Outside of the eye socket – *Which makes me feel incompetent as a pet parent.*
Under the eye – *This is all so painful and familiar—I wasn't heard as a child.*
Under the nose – *It makes me crazy.*
Under the bottom lip – *I am a bad dog person.*
Collarbone – *I can't control my dog.*
Top of the head – *It makes me sad because I don't love him like I could.*
Inside the eye socket – *If I'm totally honest with myself . . .*
Outside the eye socket – *I am always mad at my dog.*
Under the eye – *I have such deep loyalty to my other dog, Donny, who passed on two years ago.*
Under the nose – *I didn't realize how much my grief was controlling me.*
Under the bottom lip – *I am really ready to let this go—I forgive myself.*
Collarbone – *And I forgive Buddy. Buddy is just being Buddy.*
Top of the head – *In a perfect world, I have forgiven myself.*

Inside the eye socket – *I have tapped into the deep grief with Donny and am letting him go even more.*

Outside the eye socket – *I am fully accepting Buddy.*

Under the eye – *I am seeing Buddy for who he is.*

Under the nose – *I love Buddy.*

Under the bottom lip – *And because I've discovered this, we feel even more connected to each other.*

Collarbone – *We have fun and respect for each other.*

Top of the head – *We listen to each other. And we feel more in love than ever.*

For the Dog

Inside the eye socket – *When I bark, I am alerting the world that I am alive.*

Outside the eye socket – *I let everyone know what is going on!*

Under the eye – *I am letting my person/people know.*

Nose point – *I am letting the neighborhood know.*

Chin point – *You can't believe what walks by the house!*

Chest point – *My person is always on the computer.*

Top of the head – *Wow!*

Inside the eye socket – *I'm afraid they are missing out!*

Outside the eye socket – *People around me think I'm annoying.*

Under the eye – *Which makes me feel even more committed to letting them know of the dangers.*

Nose point – *I'm afraid they don't know what is going on!*

Chin point – *I actually get afraid for them!*

Chest point – *I'm afraid!*

Top of the head – *I'm afraid!*

Inside of the eye – *I'm afraid!*

Outside the eye socket – *I'm afraid that nobody will help me if one of those giant dogs out there comes into the yard.*

Under the eye – *I'm afraid that nobody's got my back.*

Nose point – *I will have to bark louder.*

Chin point – *I have to bark louder.*

Chest point – *Nobody seems to notice me.*

Top of the head – *I am trying to save our lives, for crying out loud!*

Inside the eye socket – *This is so familiar. In my first home, I was trying to save the world.*

Outside the eye socket – *Nobody noticed.*

Under the eye – *They were always mad at me.*

Nose point – *The neighbors were mad.*

Chin point – *This is so familiar.*

Chest point – *I feel like I'm in a constant battle.*

Top of the head – *A battle with the world outside the window.*

Inside the eye socket – *And a battle to help my person in distress.*

Outside the eye socket – *So clueless on the computer.*

Under the eye – *I feel like I'm not winning.*

Nose point – *And she's always so frustrated with me.*

Chin point – *Which is so familiar.*

Chest point – *So familiar.*

Top of the head – *I am so ready to try something new.*

Inside the eye socket – *I don't even know what that would be.*

Outside the eye socket – *My person doesn't seem to give a crap about what is walking by.*

Under the eye – *In fact, she shuts the door.*

Nose point – *And then I feel really lonely.*

Chin point – *I am so lonely.*

Chest point – *I am ready to try something new.*

Top of the head – *I am trying something new.*

Inside the eye socket – *I may have to just lie down in her office at her feet.*

Outside the eye socket – *I am trying something new now.*

Under the eye – *In a perfect world, I am confident.*

Nose point – *I am confident.*

Chin point – *I am confident.*

Chest point – *I am confident.*

Top of the head – *I am strong.*

Inside the eye socket – *I would rather be cozy in her office.*

Outside the eye socket – *I would rather be close to her.*

Under the eye – *We would feel so great together.*
Nose point – *We would feel cozy when she is working.*
Chin point – *We would face adventure together.*
Chest point – *I would trust her.*
Top of the head – *She would trust me. Together we are safe.*

Congratulations! You have learned the tapping sequences for humans and for all your four-legged friends. It was a lot of information to absorb, but you will soon learn that it was worth the effort. In the following chapters, you will learn how to apply the sequences to a variety of emotions, conditions, situations, and behaviors. I will also show you, through examples, the powerful shifts that can happen when you combine tapping and words with intention.

Part Two

Solutions

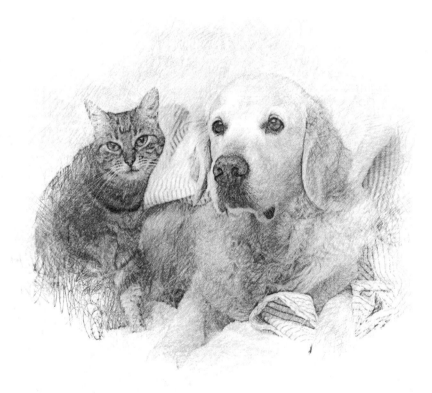

5

Emotions

This section of the book is not for the people who live with well-balanced, self-soothing and confident animals. We will explore the more challenging emotions here before we move on to behaviors, relationships/dynamics, wellness, and end of life. Also, bear in mind that there is no cookie cutter answer. All animals are individuals, and we should celebrate and work with that.

The Nature of Emotions

Emotions can be fluid. Emotions can be complex. Emotions are unique. No two beings will experience the exact same event the exact same way. Our individual emotions are as distinctive as our thumb print. Something that terrifies one puppy has zero significance for another puppy in the same litter.

Yet, one event can alter the personality of an animal, one event can inform the behavior of an animal, one event can change the trajectory of an animal, one event can alter the health of an animal. Emotions truly live in the body, mind and spirit of all animals.

Sometimes, there are secondary emotions. Sometimes, there are momentary feelings. Feelings are like ocean waves; they come and go. Feelings are driven by thought; whereas, emotions tend to drive behavior. Emotions live in the brain. The limbic system is the control center of brain function that oversees all of it.

The limbic system controls:

- Emotional responses
- Fight, flight, fright, or freeze
- Memory
- Hormones
- Attention and learning
- Reward/motivation/addictive behavior

Our animal companions are always articulating their emotional experience. Unfortunately, unless we speak dog, horse, dog, cat or domestic bird, often it is like trying to understand someone speaking very passionately in Italian when you have no understanding of the romance languages. As our companions continue to express with no result or release, this emotion becomes a neural pathway, a behavior, a pattern, a well-trodden road that they are going to trot down, regardless of whether they get in trouble for it. Or worse, they shut down.

Ultimately, why should they be in trouble due to their form of expression? Why aren't we taking the time to discover how simply they express their feelings? If we catch it early on, we might be able to avoid it turning into that universal scream, involving peeing, barking, digging, scratching, bucking over their displeasure, discomfort, discombobulation, as a result of their disempowering situation.

We tend to make their behavior wrong because it doesn't fit our lifestyle or we haven't taken the time to understand their species-specific lexicon. This compounding challenge of "inappropriate behavior" leads to animals becoming disposable. But I digress.

Knowing that the emotions are part of the body (brain/limbic system) helps us understand how an emotional situation can become a physical condition very quickly. We need to help balance the emotional life of an animal in the same way that we would tend to a wound or a broken leg. The psychology very quickly becomes the pathology for an animal, and because animals don't have the same form of expression as we do, we don't recognize their form of expression until it is often too late.

I always say that unless you have a good animal communicator, emotions are trapped in the animal's body. Certainly, time plays a role in this—over time, an animal may relax. But for lasting change, or an opportunity to help an emotional/traumatized animal, you really need the assistance of:

- A qualified, neutral animal communicator
- A seasoned animal bodyworker (such as a massage therapist, acupressure practitioner, Tellington TTouch practitioner, or craniosacral therapist)
- A truly grounded energy healer
- A gifted trainer who can get deep-seated emotions released
- An integrative, holistic and/or homeopathic veterinarian

Sometimes it's worth working with all of these special practitioners together! EFT is an energetic form of bodywork with a communication aspect. It is the most wonderful go-to for helping to release the emotions that underlie physical and behavioral challenges.

A Lasting Change

As we embark upon this Emotional Freedom Technique tapping journey, it is important to remember that no one modality is going to offer a magic pill to healing and therefore, to approach things in a holistic way. Nor would we want any short cuts. Understanding the challenge down to the core issue, or origin, of trauma helps us help our animals. It becomes part of the evolution of the relationship between you and your animal. And even when we think we are facilitating healing for another, we always get the borrowed benefit of a little healing coming our way.

It is good to support our animal companions fully on the healing journey. When working with EFT for our animals, a few ideas come to mind:

- Diet is a key factor in the physiological world that would feed the emotions (and the emotions feed the physiological).
- Other health practitioners are going to help us see the challenge through to the best result.
- Trainers and behaviorists who are on board with alternative methods are going to help make this an efficient experience. If the client can also bring on a trainer at this time and create new behaviors around an emotional experience, the animal has a much better chance of literally "rewiring" their brain. Going back to the limbic system: As we are helping the animal's brain form new memories, the limbic system helps the body learn and remember the information. It will also regulate the hormones involved, thereby making the new experience a "feel-good" event.

Entangled Feelings and Emotions

Feelings and emotions become so entangled in animals, including the human animal. When we've had an experience, we often jump from feeling to feeling to feeling. These are the subtle things we want to observe and capture if we can, in order to be able to play it back and dissolve it through EFT.

Take, for example, a young man who has the lead in the school play. For weeks before the audition, he has prepared, and he gets the role. Rehearsals are so fun. Finally, his other classmates see exactly who he is! At home, all he can talk about is his character, how much he loves his costume, his lines, the other kids in the show. He relishes the entire experience; he is in his glory.

On the big night, he is standing proud. He is ready. And then, suddenly, when he is backstage, waiting to go on stage, he hears his parents talking in the crowd, and his excitement turns to nerves and all of the blood drains from his head. His ability to function, let alone get onstage and perform the play as that character, has been hijacked. Suddenly, everything he knew has gone out the window, and his excitement has turned to nerves, panic, and freeze.

That is how fast it can happen for animals. An animal can be so excited, but it can turn from excitement to nerves to activation in a "New York minute." Sometimes, these feelings just feed each other and create a big old pattern.

Aside from our individual entangling feelings and emotions, we also tend to entangle our feelings and emotions *with* our animal companions' feelings and emotions. This is a hazardous habit of enmeshment.

When we assume that our animal companion is picking up on our panic, our fear, our anxiety, our grief, we are not seeing them as their own being with their own emotional life. This is the height of anthropocentrism, making it all about us. While they may be picking up on our feelings, they often have their own feelings of panic, fear, worry, anxiety and/or grief.

Olivia

If you've read any of my books, you will remember that I had a dog named Olivia. She was one-half Border collie, one-quarter German Shepherd, one-quarter Rottweiler, and 100 percent Scorpio. She and my cat Alexandria went through a lot with me.

I got her when I was married, but my husband and I were the victims of a heinous crime, my mother died, and we divorced. Like me, Olivia was very attached to my stepkids (okay, I'll admit, we were attached to the husband, too). It was hard for her when, all of a sudden, this family was gone. She loved rounding us all up. We all grieved—me, the dog, and the cat. But then we moved to Seattle and started a farm/healing center, and everyone began to feel better.

Then we had another setback: Alexandria disappeared. After a while Olivia and I added another dog to the family, and two years after the cat disappeared, I ended up adopting a cat that was pregnant. Several kittens later, we had a very full house again.

Then my father died. As you can imagine as I unfold this story, it was a tragic time for me. Within five years, I had lost both my parents, gotten divorced, and lost my beloved cat and stepchildren, as well as moving across the country. I was bereft, and the magnitude of it all was crushing.

In the middle of this, I injured my neck and was forced to lie on the couch (one of my favorite hobbies). While I was pretty much immobilized, I was able to observe the whole sequence of events as a pattern and realized that I had the opportunity to truly, deeply process the huge amount of grief I felt.

Olivia was grieving, too, but I told her repeatedly: "This grief is mine. You get to be the dog. I need you to be the dog now."

I frequently placed a little white bubble around Olivia and a separate bubble around me as a way of separating our fields. We were soul mates and partners in the household, yet also autonomous individual beings capable of having separate emotions and different experiences. I did not need her to take on my stuff!

I relate this story to show that I understand that life can be a rocky emotional road that sometimes feels overwhelming. I totally get how we can easily become enmeshed.

If I didn't do what I do for a living, I may have accidentally allowed her to grieve something she didn't have to.

Somehow, even in my grief, I knew I had to take on the role of emotional leader in my animal family; that it was up to me to guide Olivia to be the joy, the fun police, and all of the other glorious jobs she had in our home, and get me out into nature and, literally, smelling the roses again.

If we associate our animal's experience as only coming from us, we are never getting to the core of their feelings/emotions; therefore, anytime we or other members of the household are having an emotional experience, we trigger them continually as a result of our own codependence. Long term, this is not good for the animal's adrenal system. Ultimately, we are not helping them to heal and live in a state of confidence and independence. When we and our animal have gone through a traumatic experience together, we have even more entangled feelings and emotions, but through the process we are about to learn, we can unwind and rewind a new experience!

By breaking down some of these situations or stories and finding the main emotion or feeling, great EFT tapping scripts can emerge.

Panic

Panic swirls up as a sudden, uncontrollable fear or anxiety, often causing wild, thoughtless behavior, where we literally go blank. I have a theory about our quadrupedal friends: When they go into panic/fear/anxiety, often they become two front legs and a head. Meaning, when they are panicked, they leave their body and function from the shoulders forward; they are not necessarily thinking. A horse will swing its butt around as if it isn't even attached. Dogs tuck their tails. And cats become hovercrafts. Their forelegs become a powerful force of nature.

Panic shows up in fight or flight, mostly flight. The animal feels a total loss of control. If we were close enough, we would see a change in breathing, their heart pounding through their chest, and they may dig their toenails into our leg and shake. They may also shed, lick, dig, shred, and poop or pee. Destructive behavior is part of the panic state.

The very first experience an animal has of panic is when it is separated from its mother. This could be a repeated occurrence if a mother goes off to do something else. If a mama cat wants to go hunt, her kittens may have episodes of panic. When animals are weaned, this creates a panic that can turn to grief and/or depression.

Panic can come from being a very sensitive being, stress, chemical imbalance, a traumatic event, an accident, and of course, genetics can play a role in this. Other causes would be an emotional attachment, lack of socialization, neurological issue, or a history of abuse or neglect.

Prolonged repetitive stress can create adrenal fatigue. This lowers immunity and creates an ongoing sense of *meh!* toward everything around us. The vibrant energy just isn't there. That combination of no energy and lower immune system leaves the animal vulnerable to other diseases and/or conditions. When you have an animal that goes into a tail-spinning panic, tapping on points on good days, with or without words, helps the animal remember how to be calm. In Part One, we reviewed each of the tapping points, which are all calming and soothing. By getting your animal used to tapping, in general, you can often "get a hold of them" again when they seem to pop right out of their dog/cat/horse body in a panic.

Trauma

Trauma is not an emotion, per se, but a traumatic event creates an emotional response, and PTSD (Post Traumatic Stress Disorder) can arise. Animals that have been traumatized exhibit fearful/anxious responses to certain experiences or are completely shut down.

Neglect, abuse, and abandonment are all ways in which an animal may feel traumatized. Surgery, rehoming, or an accident may also cause trauma, as well as early socialization that has not gone well or being attacked at a young age by a littermate or by another animal later in life.

A perfect example of trauma is the animal shelter. Animals that have been dumped are traumatized because of the abandonment. Sometimes they become reactive; other times they are shut down in grief.

Fear, anxiety, grief, and rage may stand on their own and have their own origin but are often the expression of panic and/or trauma.

Fear

Fear is easily the most unpleasant emotion. It creeps in emotionally and physically, based on a belief that there is a threat or danger and may involve physical pain.

We can see it in our animals because they will start to shake, pant (breathe differently), and if you are physically close to the animal, you may even feel their heart racing. We also become aware that our animals are afraid when they either run off or screech to a halt.

For some animals, human animals included, fear takes on a life of its own. It is usually caused by an animal's personal experience sometime in the past. For some animals, such as feral cats or wild horses that end up in domestic situations, feelings of fear can go all the way back to the womb, when they gestated inside a mother who feared humans and other things. Finally, some animals are just suspicious, not confident or grounded, and have a fear of the unknown.

How Fear in the Human Body Also Impacts Our Animal Companions

As an animal communicator, I have encountered many challenges that involved a person and their animal companion experiencing a traumatic event and the human then living in fear that the situation would repeat itself and communicating that to the animal. Whether it was the person in the saddle or the person holding a leash, I knew that the human's nervous system would say all there was to say about the situation. This would be translated through the hand holding the leash, the hand holding horse reins, or the human's seat in the saddle.

This is why I went full speed ahead into getting certified and learning all I could about EFT in the early 2000s. At that time, I was living in Denver, Colorado and encountered clients whose issues brought up common themes around fear, and I tried tapping to alleviate them.

The first situation goes like this. A middle-aged woman has recently packed up her last kid for college and is experiencing empty nest syndrome. She is looking forward to going back to her life before raising children. The big passion from her past is horses. Because she knows that horses that have experienced many homes can be complicated, she decides to purchase a young horse, reasoning that this young horse will have no challenges. At some point early on, the woman gets bucked off or trampled and breaks a collarbone or a limb. Now she's afraid of the new love of her life, her horse.

The second situation involves someone stepping outside the home to walk their dog on the leash. The dog is sidelined by an aggressive unleashed dog and is pinned or injured in some horrific way.

I know that I helped clients like these, but those early years became my training ground for this work. The fear thing still rears its head with people. And for an animal lover, there's nothing worse than feeling fearful of an animal.

My friend Ellie Laks, founder of The Gentle Barn, had a big scare with a horse and was unable to even lead horses after that. This was a challenge because she lives at The Gentle Barn and there are three locations each filled with horses. It was heartbreaking, because it meant she wasn't as close as she had been with her beloved horse Whisper.

One day, I was at The Gentle Barn doing other healing work on a young cow called Ferdinand when Ellie asked me about tapping. It was then that she revealed her fear of horses to me, and I said, "Let's tap!"

We tapped on the fear, the sadness, and the disappointment, and ran through many emotions, coming back to the fear. We ended on how much ease and confidence she had with horses. I never thought to ask her anything about it, but about a year later she said to me:

"Joan, I was leading a horse out of the stall at the Tennessee Gentle Barn location, and my husband Jay asked, 'Hey, Ellie, when did you stop being afraid of horses?' and it was as if I had never been afraid of horses, and then I remembered our tapping."

When we go to heal our own emotions and feelings, logic can guide us to figure out how and why we got into a situation and lead us down our path to healing. But for many animals, their experience can lead to...

That Shaking, Salivating, Toenail-Digging Fear

Some animals (like people) are traumatized by something that someone else might experience and think was nothing yet it literally leaves an impact on that animal's soul. And some animals (like people) breeze through the most terrifying events possible. Either way, there are some emotions/experiences/traumas that totally overcome an animal (and us humans). We've all experienced it.

Some animals have a fear of cars, some have a fear of being away from home, some have a fear of other animals, some have a fear of loud noises, and some have a fear of people. It usually results in the fight, flight, fright, or freeze. They become a pancake and can't move. They become heavier than a dumbbell and you can't lift them. They flee so fast, you are spinning. Some animals can look cool as a cucumber with a little faraway look in their eyes and their stomach is flipping inside and out and their poop will tell the story later.

The hardest part of being an animal empath (and you wouldn't be reading this book if you weren't one, too) is that we pick up on that energy. As their guardian, it can be heartbreaking to watch our animal companions suffer and struggle. It starts out sad for the human and can then move to frustrating, as we think that the animal should get over it and feel like a failure because we should have fixed this by now.

Step one in our personal program for dealing with our animals and their fear, anxiety, timidity, and/or aggression is to stay grounded. In both of my earlier books—*Communication with All Life: Revelations of an Animal Communicator* (Hay House) and *Energy Healing for Animals* (Sounds True)—I talk about how we must be the emotional leader.

This is why we also tap on ourselves. We don't always realize how much our own being is contributing to or compounding our animal companion's situation. By tapping on ourselves first, we often release some of the pressure the animal is experiencing.

Timid

Communication with All Life University (CWALU) students are required to do case studies. They must do 65 case studies in animal communication, 65 case studies in energy healing with scalar wave, and 65 case studies in EFT. This is in addition to the classroom hours of communicating and healing and all the homework the students do with each other. By the time they leave the school, they have communicated with and facilitated healing for and with hundreds of animals.

I share this because this next story shows how one of my students, Tanya, who at the time was in the early stages of her case studies, helped an "unadoptable" dog from a rescue become integrated into the pack.

Tanya reached out to Bella, who operates a German Shepherd rescue center in Florida, and inquired about unadoptable dogs. Bella told her that she did have a dog that was unadoptable and didn't know what to do with her.

The dog, Lady, had come from a home where she had been tied up outside and neglected, essentially a bad situation all the way around. As a result, Lady was shut down, shy, nervous and didn't want to have anything to do with the other dogs in the rescue or Bella's own personal pack. Bella was afraid that she would have to keep Lady because it didn't seem possible that she could overcome these issues.

Enter tapping! When Tanya did her animal communication session, she picked up on what an old soul Lady was but that she lived in a world of anxiety and shutdown. Lady had a nervous tummy and would chomp at the air. Even though all of this was going on for Lady, and she was very timid with dogs and people, she wanted to belong.

Tanya tapped on all those feelings—the anxiety, feeling shut down, the nervous tummy, and letting go of the past. Since Lady wanted to belong, Tanya tapped with Lady about feeling safe and secure in her environment.

Then Tanya tapped with Bella. As founder of a big rescue operation, Bella is by nature a fixer. It can be very disappointing when you can't fix something! Tanya tapped with Bella about being a fixer and not being able to truly rescue this dog, even though she was safe in the rescue.

The next day Bella sent Tanya a video of what had happened after the session.

Lady had gone outside as she normally did in the morning, and instead of being completely shut down, started running around and engaging in play with the other dogs. Tanya shared the video with her fellow students, and it was totally heartwarming and fun! Lady was adopted four months later.

Fear of Strangers

"Stranger danger," as it is popularly known, falls somewhere between anxiety and straight-up fear or even abject terror. Barnaby was at abject terror level. His person, Claudia, is now one of the teachers at CWALU and an animal communicator/healer in her own right. When she began the CWALU program, I asked her to bring her dog, as she lived locally, and we needed another dog to do the healing work with.

The one problem was that there was a guy in the class. Usually, my classes are primarily women, but during this particular Spring Intensive class, there was a dude named Pete.

Now, there is nobody gentler than Pete. He exudes safety . . . to humans, that is; not to Barnaby, who was terrified of all men. Back then, I would cram about 35–45 people into a relatively small room, so there was really nowhere for Barnaby to retreat. He ended up hiding behind Claudia's chair.

We tapped on Barnaby's "stranger danger" fear and then tapped on his terror. Once that started to shift, we turned it around to such an extent that Barnaby is now Claudia's "knight in shining armor," her fearless protector.

By the Fall Intensive, Barnaby was way more chilled around people, men, and just in general. He might still bark, but he now runs up, touches the person, and runs off. Sometimes, he even relaxes in the same room as a strange guy. He is curious. Through the tapping we went from panic to seeking behavior.

Is he totally fine with strangers? No. But the terror is gone.

Fear of Sounds

Kim graduated from the CWALU program a few years back. During the energy healing portion of her curriculum, she used her own dog, Oski, as the subject not only for me to work on tapping with him in class but also for her homework partners to work with after class.

Oski was terrified of fireworks. Unfortunately for him, they lived near Disneyland in Southern California, and Disneyland has nightly fireworks. Every night, this 80-pound dog would pant, get very nervous, and try to climb into Kim's lap. Kim doesn't weigh much more than 80 pounds herself. (Okay, maybe a bit more, but she is tiny.) She does not have a lap that can fit an 80-pound dog. As she described it, "He was not in his body."

Once Kim learned more about tapping, she started tapping on him about the fireworks, soothing Oski through the experience. Oski started coming to Kim when the fireworks started so that she could soothe him by tapping on him. He loved the tapping and is no longer afraid of fireworks.

Anxiety

Anxiety gets its hooks into us physically as the mind races. It is simply the mind/body's reaction to stress, danger, unfamiliar situations, certain people, medical conditions, social situations, and being triggered by a memory. Sometimes, anxiety keeps animals alert, vigilant, but even this more subtle version isn't always great for the mind/body. Another way of saying it would be, this is a very nervous cat/horse/dog.

Anxiety can come in the form of licking, digging, shredding, and peeing in the house. It can also be extreme vigilance, shedding, pacing, panting, and weird body language. Anxiety shows up as absolute destruction, including putting themselves in a nearly suicidal position, meaning, they don't mind hurting themselves through engaging in the anxiety-ridden activity.

Sometimes, you can just sense that an animal is waiting for "the other shoe to drop." Anxiety can be internalized. The dog can seem super chill, but his potty habits let you know he is tightly wound. You might see this more in their digestion—the poop will tell the story.

Often this stems from an early trauma, maybe having to fend for food, being out on the streets, being in the shelter too long, a lack of socialization, a history of abuse, to name a few. It can also be genetic, neurological, environmental, related to emotional attachment, enmeshment, pain, and more.

Anxiety can even creep into someone who has experienced a seeming non-event, such as being in the crate when kids are playing outside. It could come from being carsick, slipping in the snow, thunder and lightning, and so much more. There is no shortage of things that could make an animal anxious!

Zip

Monkey Zip could fly around his enclosure and wow people at the prestigious zoo where he lived. But it was obvious that there was something wrong with him as he was alone, whereas every other primate area had families or communities.

Zip was stunning, elusive, and the public admired him. He had been alone in an enclosure for over a year when I met him, because he was exhibiting extreme anxiety and had been rather aggressive to the females when he was with his community. He was agitated by all the other monkeys in the enclosures around him now. He didn't necessarily love humans, either.

After communicating with him and discovering how out of control and sad he felt, I offered to do EFT on him, and the zookeeper was all for it.

We tapped on his loneliness and need to control. He never sat close to people while in the private part of the enclosure.

During the communication and EFT, he sat on the other side of the screen from me as I did surrogate tapping for him, and he soaked in every moment of it.

His personal zookeeper said that he was much calmer after that. He became more at peace with himself and the fact that he had to be alone. He was also more tolerant of the people watching him and the shenanigans of the neighboring monkeys.

Victor

A young girl, Barb, and her mother had me out to talk to her new pony, Victor. Victor was a champ! He had been imported from Germany, and Barb was thrilled. At 12 years of age, Barb seemed to be living the dream!

In the initial animal communication session, Victor told me of winning everything with his prior person, a young girl in Germany. He has a very confident professional demeanor and seemed to be adjusting well here in the US, though he was a little unsure of his job with Barb. Victor found Barb to be a little anxious. He had never felt this before, his riders in Germany were all rather confident.

Barb's mother assured me that Barb was not anxious, but months later, she called again, wanting another session. It seemed that Barb was now terrified of Victor (an understatement), after he had bolted with her. I can't remember if she had fallen off Victor, but regardless, her true fear was of Victor bolting.

When I returned to the dressage barn where Victor lived, he reiterated his confusion with his job and the fact that Barb was very nervous—all the time.

Finally, Barb's mother admitted that Barb did indeed have a severe anxiety disorder. Not only that but she was so terrified of riding Victor that she was exhibiting fear in the car ride to the barn.

I asked them if they wanted to try something weird (tapping) and suggested we go around the corner where no one could see us pounding on our own faces! I also explained this may take more than one session.

We took Victor over to a grassy spot where he could relax, and I asked Barb several things:

- *Where in her body was her terror of riding Victor?* She said it was in her stomach.
- *Did she want to get on Victor again?* She said yes.
- *Did this terror remind her of anything that had happened before?* She said she had been in a car wreck at one point. The mother said it was nothing, a fender bender. For Barb, this feeling of being out of control, trapped in a seat in the back, was beyond anything she wanted to experience again.
- *If she could ride again, who was her absolute hero?* Suddenly, this shy, seemingly anxious young girl sat up and instantly said Charlotte Dujardin and Valegro. Now I knew what we were doing, for sure. Charlotte Dujardin and Valegro are an Olympic dream. While taking part in several Olympics, they have won three gold medals and one silver medal through years together riding for the UK.

I knew I had my work cut out for me. This young girl was even wearing a helmet to the barn to groom her horse, along with a vest to protect herself, lest her horse were to get out of control. Yet, her vision of riding like Charlotte Dujardin was palpable.

This time, I started tapping with the concept that everything was "out of control, out of control." At some point, we even repeatedly tapped on the out of control on every point. I kept coming back to that. I then ended it with, "And we float, airborne, like Pegasus, a team like Charlotte Dujardin and Valegro." I consistently used the Charlotte and Valegro reference through all the points.

I also constantly checked back with her on how her stomach felt. I would throw lines into the script like, "Oh, my stomach says no, I can't get back on." I knew that this energy, defeat, fear, anxiousness, feeling of out of control was sitting in her stomach, and I could always use that as a reference point for progress.

I also tapped on Victor about feeling out of control and ended with him becoming like Valegro.

As I would feel Barb and Victor shifting, I would remind Victor, as if I were tapping into his brain, that his new job was to always take care of Barb. Then I would go into the Charlotte and Valegro imagery.

I asked Barb to have her parents take a picture of Charlotte and Valegro and put Barb's head on Charlotte's body and Victor's face on Valegro's body. Within a day or so, after the first session, Barb's parent's emailed me this brilliantly photoshopped photo of Victor's head on Valegro's body and Barb's head on Charlotte's body.

In truth, it took several sessions to make progress, but Barb had a lot of old anxiety to work through; however, it didn't take long for Victor to regain the confidence he had had as a German sport pony.

Between the tapping, Victor's confidence, and kindness, and, of course, the training Barb was undertaking, it all came together. I was so grateful to receive a holiday card with Barb riding Victor on a trail, beaming. The beautiful card sat on my table, long after the holidays, as a reminder that all things are possible.

Grief

Grief is the deepest form of sorrow, usually over the loss of a loved one. The first grief an animal feels is when their litter, herd, or pack is broken up and the other siblings go in many different directions and are weaned from their mother.

Usually, they never see their family again, and grief then becomes like a backdrop that is revisited throughout life.

Grief can also come from the death of their human or if they lose their person due to a divorce or a rehoming situation. Grief is deep within the animal family, and bonded animal family members grieve tremendously if someone dies or is rehomed.

Moving homes can cause grief. A person changing the routine can cause grief. Animals retiring from a job can cause grief. The body no longer working like it used to can cause grief. Loss of a limb can lead to grief. And grief can lead to anxiety. Grief is closely associated with sadness, and if left unchecked it can turn into depression and being shut down. This happens in no particular order.

We see it in listlessness. We see it when the light in their eyes has dimmed. We see it when they sleep a lot. Or that gregarious animal is suddenly sullen and internalizing. And sometimes, we even see tears coming from their eyes.

Rage

Rage is violent, uncontrollable anger, the kind that is red-hot and can be scary. It is way beyond being annoyed or put off, though that can build into a big reaction. For example, a puppy bugs the older dog and the older dog says no gently, says no gently again, and after the third or fourth time, the older dog snaps in a fit of anger.

We see rage through aggressive behaviors, such as protecting resources, offspring, and territory. We also see it in a quick reaction to something we are asking them to do. Sometimes it is even in response to touching an area we are unaware is hurt.

Rage can come from a chemical imbalance, neurological disorders, a past experience they will no longer tolerate, and of course, protection. We will walk through rage in many of the forms of aggression we will be working on in Chapter 6.

Tapping on Emotions

In the next few chapters, we will be addressing specific behaviors, dynamics, conditions, wellness/health challenges, and end of life in your animal. I will break down the scripts for each of these specific issues then, but if you want to tap on some of these very big and deep emotions before then, let me guide you through this with the following sample investigation, both for yourself and your animal.

As noted earlier, I like to set an intention for what I am tapping on for the animal. For example: "I'd love for her to feel peace." "I'd love for him to feel confident." "I'd love for us to be closer." Before you start the investigation, really think through what a perfect outcome would be.

Remember, even if this animal is new to you, your nervous system is going to be contributing to their situation, so being grounded and neutral or willing to tap on yourself is advised. Even a brand-new animal to you in a compromised situation, such as being shut down, full of rage, anxious, and so forth, could quickly bring up feelings in you, such as:

- I feel helpless.
- I feel frustrated.
- I feel angry that someone could do this to this animal.
- I feel distraught.

And if it is your own animal, you may be adding thoughts like:

- I feel like a terrible guardian.
- I'm so sad for them when they hurt like this.
- I can't believe that I'm so triggered by this.
- I can't believe I let it get to this point.
- I have so much guilt.

We are always leading to the animal feeling:

- Safe
- Grounded
- Confident
- Happy
- Loved
- Full of joy

Let's Tap

The following is how I like to get started with tapping. Note: This tapping template is repeated in the Appendix, where it can be easily copied and used for reference.

Grounding

Personally, I meditate daily and have a practice of using my other favorite technique, the Scalar Wave, on myself to ground my energy first thing in the morning. If I am tapping on an animal in person, I like to help them get grounded as well. I may just sit and take some deep breaths with them to calm them and try to match our breathing.

I might do something called the Bladder Sweep, which is a physical sweep down the bladder meridian. As we know from the first tapping point on the face, that is Bladder 1, the start of the Bladder meridian. It runs parallel to the spine, down the hind legs to the outside toe on both hind legs. I would stroke three times from the top of their head down to the left hind outside toe, then three times from the top of their head down to the right outside toe, then three times from the top of the head to the end of the tail. If they are missing a limb or the tail, I still do it to the phantom limb or tail.

Review

I like to review what the circumstances are, whether it is a relationship dynamic or an event that is causing the present reality.

I take the script (see farther down) and investigate *my own feelings (or those of the human I'm working with)* and take copious notes. While there may be a story as a framework for the situation, these notes largely identify several feelings and emotions involved in the current state.

I take the script and investigate *the animal's feelings* based on either an animal communication session or what would very clearly be the feelings for the animal based on their behavior, and again take copious notes. While there may be a story as a framework for the situation, these notes largely identify several feelings and emotions involved in the current state.

Intention

What is it I'm trying to accomplish here? What is my intention? Is it peace? Well-being? Getting clear on the intention is vital for a desired outcome.

Outcome

What is the final outcome? This is something worth spending time on at the end of the tapping, either by tapping several rounds or creating a visualization for you and your animal of the desired outcome for both (or all) beings. Even if the animal is going to transition (to a new home, a new job or the eternal home) have a peaceful vision like a guided meditation that you are able to say out loud and feel the joy, peace or relief that this can offer. All beings want safety and security above all else. Ending with the animal feeling safe, confident and feeling good in their own skin is also a wonderful outcome.

Sample Script – Investigation for the Human

Karate Chop point setup statement:

- *Round 1*: Share the story of what happened and your emotions around the experience, and end with "And I love and accept myself."
- *Round 2*: Share more of your story and your big emotions around the event or relationship, and end with "And I fully accept myself."
- *Round 3*: Share how this animal's big emotions continue to trigger you and end with "I honor the choices I'm making."

Inside eye socket: *When this happened* ....

....

OR

When my animal ....

Outside eye socket: *I feel* ....

....

Under eye: *I also feel* ....

....

Under nose: *I continue to feel* ....

....

Chin: *People around me think* ....

....

Collarbone: *Which makes me feel even more* ....

....

Pick one of the following:

Top of head: *If I'm honest, I may be getting a secondary gain of* ....

....

It's familiar and reminds me of ....

....

Pick one of the following transition setups:

Inside eye socket: *I am feeling blocked/resistant to shift/I'm in a big battle, because* ....

....

....

I struggle with my deep-seated belief/vow/loyalty to my feelings, because ....

....

Big Forgiveness or Letting-Go Transition Statement

Pick one of the following:

Outside eye socket: *I forgive myself. I am ready to let this go.*

It's time to move on.

I'm ready to try something new.

I can't take it anymore.

Under eye: *In a perfect world my animal companion would* ....

....

....

Under nose: *And we would feel* ....

....

....

NOTE: If a big feeling doesn't seem to release, don't hesitate to tap several rounds (through all of the points) just on that one emotion or feeling.

Sample Script – Investigation for the Animal

Inside eye socket: *When I feel* ....

....

OR

when .... *happens*

Outside eye socket: *I feel* ....

....

Under the eye: *I also feel* ....

Top of the nose: *I continue to feel* ....

....

Under the chin: *People around me think* ....

....

Collarbone: *Which makes me feel even more* ....

....

Pick one of the following:

Top of head: *If I'm honest, I may be getting a secondary gain of* ....

....

....

It's familiar and reminds me of ....

....

Pick one of the following:

Top of head: *If I'm honest, I may be getting a secondary gain of* ....

....

It's familiar and reminds me of...

....

Pick one of the following:

Top of head: *If I'm honest, I may be getting a secondary gain of* ....

....

It's familiar and reminds me of...

....

Pick one of the following transition setups:

Inside the eye socket: *I am feeling blocked/resistant to shift/I'm in a*

big battle, because ....

....

I struggle with my deep-seated belief/vow/loyalty to my feelings, because

....

Big Forgiveness or Letting-Go Transition Statement

Pick one of the following:

Outside eye socket: *I forgive myself. I am ready to let this go* (statement
can be reversed).

It's time to move on.

I'm ready to try something new.

I can't take it anymore.

Top of the nose: *In a perfect world my person and I would* ....

....

Under the chin: *And we would feel* ....

....

NOTE: If a big feeling doesn't seem to release, don't hesitate to tap
several rounds (through all of the points) just on that one emotion or
feeling.

6

Behavior

Before we jump into behaviors of animals that are emotion-based, remember just that: These are emotion-based behaviors; therefore, they can be trained out, conditioned out, healed out of them. Nobody is any one thing all the time, not even the meanest junkyard dog.

Other behaviors could stem from medical conditions. For example, seizures could bring on rage syndrome or anxiety, and thyroid issues can bring on unwanted behavior. If you think that the behavior that your animal exhibits is much deeper than emotional, it is best to consult with a veterinarian, particularly, a holistic veterinarian.

While I am holistically minded, and prefer all things energetic, herbal, mineral, plant-based or homeopathic, if the behavior is deeply embedded, some sort of medication short term to retrain the neural pathway is not the worst idea to add to this protocol. If you are working with a holistic vet, you may be able to manage things by using supplements, herbs, homeopathy, or flower essences without resorting to chemicals.

This is not meant to be a paint-by-numbers kit; rather, it is an examination of whether or not your animal fits in a particular category, and if not, try another one.

In the meantime, always be willing to seek outside help. A great trainer, behaviorist, and/or holistic veterinarian who is open (even if they are not) may be the best support you can have on this journey. And remember, it is a journey. This behavior didn't happen overnight; therefore, it may take some unraveling from a few angles.

Aggression aka Reactivity

Aggression is hostile, threatening, or violent behavior toward another being—standing ground with a hostile attitude and a readiness to attack or confront. Sometimes it is provoked, and sometimes it appears to come out of nowhere. Of course, it always comes from somewhere; it's a matter of finding where it came from.

Aggression can be scary for the human if they don't know where the jolt of anger in the animal came from. It can be bigger than life, shocking, and can bring up a lot of sadness for both the human and the animal. Unless the animal is treated for it, it is like being hostage to a behavior. Often this requires a diagnosis from an animal behaviorist or a respected trainer who is well versed in the subject of aggression.

Reactivity, on the other hand, can look like a moment of aggression. While the reaction in the moment can seem aggressive, even angry, the underlying cause may be fear, lack of socialization, pain, overstimulation, and so on—it often isn't anger at all. If unchecked, reactivity can escalate into aggression.

With a very broad brushstroke, we will break down many of the types of animal reactivity/aggressions. By no means is this a behavior diagnosis, and if you are experiencing something big at home with your animal—something that is somewhere between aggression and reactivity, and you aren't sure what it is—it is always best to consult with a professional.

Aggression is a wide-ranging subject. There are over 21 possible types of aggression in dogs, yet there are common threads throughout.

For example, many people think that their dog is protecting them when, in truth, it is not; it is protecting itself, because it doesn't feel the emotional leadership from its human. Many people think that their animal has been abused when, in truth, its aggression may have come from an overall fear. Some people think their animal is crazy, when maybe they don't understand the external stimulus. Some people really get their feelings hurt when they don't know that the animal is feeling pain or protecting an old wound.

Fear-Based Reactivity/Aggression in Dogs

- **Control Conflict Reactivity/Aggression** – The dog needs control over its environment.
- **Fear Reactivity/Aggression** – This starts as threatening behavior and often the dog retreats.
- **Neophobia** – The dog is afraid of new situations, new people, new everything.
- **Leash Reactivity/Aggression** – This can start with a lot of excitable barking, which turns to nervous barking then lunging, biting, growling.

Protection Reactivity/Aggression in Dogs

- **Protective Reactivity/Aggression** – When a third party approaches, these dogs protect their person.
- **Territorial Reactivity/Aggression** – If an intruder comes into the area, they are in deep trouble with this dog.
- **Learned Reactivity/Aggression** – The dog is protective over toys and more and has learned that snapping gets what it wants.
- **Maternal Reactivity/Aggression** – This dog is protective of its litter and itself. Things usually return to normal when the dog's hormones rebalance or puppies are weaned.
- **Dominance** – This dog thinks it is the alpha dog of the pack, bossing other dogs and sometimes people. This is a dog that feels he must prove himself.
- **Dog-on-Dog Reactivity/Aggression** – This dog demonstrates consistently aggressive responses to other dogs in the absence of a threat.
- **Possessive Reactivity/Aggression** – These dogs are protective of high-value items like toys, food, or other resources.

Physical or Pain-Related Reactivity/Aggression in Dogs

- **Pain-related Reactivity/Aggression** – These dogs may be protective of old injuries, post-op, and/or painful parts of themselves, past pain, and "muscle memory." These are often triggered when you go to pick them up.
- **Idiopathic Aggression** – This is rage syndrome, often from a neurological or seizure-related disease or severe attack. Afterwards, they look confused.
- **Hypothyroidism** – The dog's thyroid gland is underperforming leading to reactivity behavior. Thyroid medication often reverses this within a week.
- **Head Injuries** – Dogs with head injuries are often reactive.

Outer, Over, or Zero Stimulation

- **Predatory Reactivity/Aggression** – The prey instinct is switched on in these dogs, and they may chase small animals, bicyclists, and children running past.
- **Redirecting Reactivity/Aggression** – This is where aggression gets retargeted at someone or something new if the dog can't get to the thing it is chasing. The dog experiences pent-up frustration, largely due to being on a leash or being cooped up behind a fence and having no release.

Cats have Reactivity/Aggression, Too!

I can't imagine a cat having FOMO (fear of missing out), but if they ever did, it would be about being left out of the aggression discussion!

Fear-Based Reactivity/Aggression in Cats

- **Fear Aggression** – This starts out as fear of the unknown, but after a big hiss, they retreat.

Protection Reactivity/Aggression in Cats

- **Play/Predatory** – This usually starts out as play, turns to stalking, then takes a turn for the striking attack.
  Maternal Reactivity/Aggression – The mother cat is protective of her babies and herself. This usually returns to normal when hormones rebalance or the kittens are weaned.
- **Cat-on-Cat Reactivity/Aggression** – This behavior is usually territorial, though could be from a bad experience early in life.

Physical or Pain-Related Reactivity/Aggression in Cats

- **Pain-Induced Reactivity/Aggression** – Sometimes animals are protective of old injuries, post-op, and/or painful parts of themselves, past pain, and "muscle memory," which is often triggered when you go to pick them up.

Outer, Over, or Zero Stimulation in Cats

Petting-Induced Reactivity/Aggression – Cats aren't as social as dogs. They may groom each other, but they are independent. There is an "overstimulation" button on most cats, and they will give subtle cues several times before they attack.
- **Redirected Reactivity/Aggression** – This is pent-up frustration, largely due to being bored.

Any of these forms of aggression could come from boredom, learned behavior, abandonment, lack of socialization, genetic, lack of exercise, lack of emotional leadership, trauma, deep grief, extreme loss, chaotic start, and many, many more possibilities as to why this would have an impact and the cat react through aggression. We can add to this, kittens born to a feral mother, which literally picked up the fear, panic, and protective sense from the mother while in utero.

Horses Can Be Reactive/Aggressive

Horses can be reactive/aggressive as well. How do they show aggression? If you've ever been standing there and witnessed in the distance a horse coming full force, straight at you, and you don't know if it is safe to jump left or right, you have just met horse reactivity. A freight train rumbling down the tracks would be easier to avoid!

Biting, kicking, pushing, charging, bucking, rearing, bolting (think rocket being blasted into space), and of course, pinning back their ears and going after another horse, human, or dog are all very clear examples of reactive/aggressive behavior in horses.

Fear-Based Reactivity/Aggression in Horses

- **Fear** – This starts as threatening behavior, with ears pinned back, maybe some teeth bared, and certainly a toss of the head, and often the horse then retreats.
- **Dominance** – As a habit, horses with this tendency lean on the person, literally, as if they could get in your pocket. This stems from a need for both protection and/or attention and is a very dangerous habit.

Protection Reactivity/Aggression in Horses

- **Resource/Territorial/Dominance** – We've all seen the stallion among the wild herd. He is the guy who will make sure that he maintains his resources (food and mares), his territory, and he does it through a dominant stance.

Pain-Related Reactivity/Aggression in Horses

- **Chronic Pain** – This is the horse that makes biting motions at you when you cinch the saddle and bucks when you ask them to canter in a particular direction to avoid pain in a hip that isn't working right.
- **Association with Previous Pain** – This is a response to past pain. Even though in the present moment the spot may not "hurt," the horse experiences muscle memory of pain there.

Outer, Over, or Zero Stimulation in Horses

- **Bucking, Rearing, and/or Bolting** – A horse might have been slowly grazing and ambling for two-thirds of the day and then react, possibly due to lack of exercise and understimulation.

- **Bucking, rearing and/or bolting** – Conversely, this behavior can also indicate overstimulation.

Domestic Birds

What makes a domestic bird become aggressive/reactive? While I can't pretend to be a bird specialist, and birds made up a small fraction of my practice as an animal communicator over the years, I did see some significant behaviors and they have similar underlying circumstances that might create the behavior.

Fear-Based Reactivity/Aggression in Birds

- Fear
- Lack of socialization
- Hadn't been hand-fed as a baby
- Old trauma
- Born in the wild

Protection Reactivity/Aggression in Birds

- Protective of their cage
- Perch protection – sometimes seen as dominance
- Seeing one human as their bonded pair and not wanting others around
- Possessive over other birds

Pain-Related Reactivity/Aggression in Birds

- Hormones in younger birds
- Protecting an injury

Outer, Over, or Zero Stimulation in Birds

- Boredom
- Frustration
- Not socialized

Any of these forms of aggression could come from learned behavior, abandonment, lack of socialization, genetic, lack of exercise, lack of emotional leadership, trauma, deep grief, extreme loss, chaotic start to life, and many, many more possibilities as to why this would have an impact and the animal would react through reactivity/aggression. Sometimes, reactivity/aggression comes from bad habits formed early on, such as orphaned colts, puppies, or kittens that have been abandoned by their mom.

Breaking It Down

When going through the EFT discovery process for any of these situations, start by trying to understand or intuit why the animal has become reactive/aggressive, then seek to understand the emotions behind it for the animal: fear, panic, confusion, threatened, overstimulation, boredom, and so forth.

For the human, these behaviors can be overwhelming, sad, frustrating, and maddening, and you can feel like a hostage to your own animal and their situation. If you are the go-to animal person in the neighborhood and your animal has a reactivity/aggression issue, it can be quite embarrassing.

Exuberance Gone Awry

I have a term for some forms of leash reactivity/aggression: "leash exuberance." I have seen it time and time again and experienced it with my own dog, Delilah. When it happened with my own dog, I had already worked with hundreds, if not thousands, of people with this challenge, so when faced with it myself, I broke it down, second by second.

Delilah is a Border Collie cross and Sagittarius party girl and loves to play. She is happiest when she is surrounded by those she loves (dogs, humans, or cats) and offers little quick licks and kisses to remind you of how big she loves. She always has a smile on her face.

Delilah was raised by two older dog siblings. Olivia (one-half Border Collie, one-quarter German Shepherd, one-quarter Rottweiler, and 100 percent Scorpio) was about 10 years old when Delilah was adopted, and Isabella (supermodel Black Lab and Libra) was roughly six years old. They all played hard and loved hard. Weekly, we would go on a large pack walk with a student of mine who is a dog trainer. We, the humans, would be in a sea of canines, sometimes up to 17 dogs, including my three. Each week, Delilah was introduced to several new dogs and the old standbys. My dogs lived for Tuesdays.

When Delilah was about four years old we moved to California, and within a year, we lost both Olivia and Isabella. We adopted Abby (a Black Lab/Shar Pei cross and Libra) between those two losses. While we had some dog friends here and there, we weren't in large packs anymore.

One day, I took my dogs to the beach. When I got out of the car, I had to put my dogs on leashes. As we walked the trail to get to the beach, Delilah was getting more and more excited, as she loved the beach. But then, to my shock, as we passed other dogs, Delilah became unglued barking and raging at them. She went from zero to 60 in a nano-second. It took every ounce of my strength to keep Delilah with me, and I handle horses daily.

Meanwhile, Abby was unfazed. She is as beta as it gets and beats to her own drummer. So I have one dog to the left of me completely unhinged and Abby hoping for a scent tour. I had never seen this behavior—or so I thought.

I chalked it up to the fact that we hadn't been to the beach since Isabella died and Delilah was excited, but it kept on happening, so I had to gear up to go anywhere.

I tapped with her a bit but at first, I was so shocked by the behavior, I wasn't as committed as I should have been to healing this as I didn't really understand it. It was so big, so overwhelming, that I couldn't even picture her walking by a dog without reacting. That's when I knew I needed help, because I can visualize just about anything and this felt like unknown territory!

Eventually, I decided to work with a trainer, Stefano Filippelli; he took one of my animal communication classes. Stefano asked me some key questions, and we broke it down slowly.

Here I am, the one who talks about Emotional Leadership in both of my previous books, and it had not occurred to me that I was not the emotional leader for Delilah. Essentially, I had allowed Olivia and Isabella to raise her, and while neither of those older dogs were ever reactive, they *were* protective of our old farm.

I got clear on two things: first, I was not being an emotional leader for Delilah and needed some training, and second, without that leadership, Delilah remained confused, scared, and honestly, didn't know how to be. This clarity helped me so much. Even though it looked scary as hell, she was simply reacting to all of the above.

For Delilah, I tapped on her loss of Olivia and Isabella as leaders, her confusion, her fear, and her needing protection. For myself, I tapped on my guilt for being a bad emotional leader, my sadness that she was trapped like this in a life of reactivity, my shock that I have a dog like this, and just in general, what a bad dog person I must be.

I am happy to say between the tapping and work with Stefano, we can pass just about any situation without her giving it a second thought. If I see her assuming the position of blastoff into reactivity, I simply say, "Leave it!"

Kim and Oski

Let's revisit Kim and Oski from Chapter 5. Kim graduated from the CWALU program a few years back. During the energy healing portion of her curriculum, she used her own dog Oski as the subject for not only class where I got to tap with him but also with her homework partners. In Chapter 5, we discussed his fear of loud noises, but here, we will share more.

Oski had what Kim considered "leash aggression" on walks. It sounded very much like the "leash exuberance" I had experienced with Delilah. When we broke down each moment in class, it was similar to what I had experienced: Oski was excited to go out, but once out, he became nervous around certain dogs, and the lunging and snarling would begin.

"I want to enjoy walking with my dog," Kim said.

But that was the last thing she was experiencing. Ever vigilant, she had to remain watchful about every dog coming around a corner, because it wasn't every dog that caused a reaction in Oski; it was only certain dogs. Her husband couldn't control Oski at all. As a result of Kim being the police essentially, she wasn't enjoying her dog as much.

In the initial EFT inquiry, we discovered that Oski didn't feel safe—so simple, yet that was the last thing Kim or her husband would have suspected based on what seemed to be very aggressive behavior. Once we tapped on that and all the feelings that Kim had, such as guilt over not picking up on the fear and how frustrated she was with Oski, a whole lot was released.

Now, Kim enjoys her walks with Oski, and so does her husband. Oski doesn't have to worry anymore—he is free to just be the ever-sniffing dog.

Kim says, "Now he is fine. He doesn't instigate anything, and if there is any sort of a moment, I can calm him."

Aggression with Humans

One of the scarier things on the planet is to feel like an animal has turned on you. Just as scary is to watch your animal do everything in its power to shred someone.

When I was first called to communicate with Spike, a noble German Shepherd, I had no idea of the careers his humans, Anna and Dave, were involved in. Spike shared with me that Anna (his human) had a deep need for security, and he took it upon himself to take care of her. Delving deeper, I learned that both of Anna's parents, and she herself, had been in the military and she was compulsive about locking doors and watching every move a stranger might make.

Anna had left a fancy Homeland Security job in Washington, DC to marry a man she loved, Dave, a sheriff in Dallas, Texas. She had secured other work in Dallas and moved in with Dave, and Spike was included in the marriage package.

Unfortunately, Spike was cornering Dave in his own house when he walked in from work. The garage was on the bottom level of a three-story house, and every day, when Dave came home, he was cornered in the basement until Anna had coaxed Spike away from Dave. Once Dave was upstairs, they were able to enjoy watching movies together on the couch and relaxing moments.

After the communication, and Anna revealing how correct Spike was (she needed extra security and support), I knew what to tap on. With Spike, we tapped on his devotion, loyalty, and need for control. We also tapped on his confusion about his new role in this household. With Anna, we tapped on her deep-seated need for security and how difficult it was to transition into the unknown, even though she loved Dave.

Dave claims that he wasn't scared, just irritated by Spike's behavior. Maybe Dave is that tough or sensed that Spike was never going to do anything. Either way, Dave agreed to tap.

In the end, Dave was able to get out of his car and come upstairs without being under siege by threat of the pearly whites of a German Shepherd. Being able to relax in his own home on all three floors was a nice reprieve for Dave and certainly a relief for how the marriage would go in Anna's mind.

Peeing/Marking and More

This is another big topic. Humans have little rooms to pee in. We take all kinds of sanitary precautions afterward, and "EMPLOYEES, WASH YOUR HANDS" signs can be seen in movie theaters, grocery stores, and other places. Nowhere on a tree (or lamppost) will you find a similar sign for animals. For them, peeing is a whole different story—literally, it tells a story, as for many animals, peeing is a way of communicating. Our dogs wake up to read their "peemail." Because their olfactory sense is anywhere from 10,000–100,000 times more acute than ours, their "smeller" tells them everything they need to know about other animals.

Cats not only communicate through scent but see the blending of scents involved in peeing in certain spots as potentially bonding. Because we don't entirely understand the world of cat pee, we once again measure it through the lens of our human world, where peeing outside of the toilet is typically seen as gross.

If it isn't marking, it could be peeing due to an emotional or physical issue, lack of training, excitement, and/or submissive peeing. When we measure animals by our standards of peeing, we are missing the story.

If I noticed mysterious peeing taking place, I would start by checking if my dog or cat had anything going on that would fit into one of the following four categories:

- **Marking/Spraying** – territorial
- **Emotional** – straight-up emotional if not a training malfunction
- **Physical** – UTI's, kidney/bladder disease, idiopathic cystitis, and more
- **Overstimulation Resulting in Excitement/Submissive Peeing** – peeing for opposite reasons

Sometimes, it is a combination of all of the above based on habit, because it wasn't dealt with early on.

Marking/Spraying

The conversation with the client always goes like this: "I can't tell if it is marking [dog] or spraying [cat] versus just plain peeing."

There are a few things to consider when it comes to marking/spraying versus peeing in a dog or cat. One way to tell which it is (but don't count on this) is that marking/spraying is generally on a vertical surface while peeing is on a horizontal surface.

Marking can be a way of saying "I am not safe." Whether you are a dog or a cat, if a new animal in the neighborhood or even new to your household is swinging by, that is upsetting to your animal's routine, even downright threatening. Maybe there's a new human in the picture, or some other big change. Marking a new house is an efficient way for your dog or cat to feel right at home! Nothing says "Welcome!" better than adding their own unique scent decoration (followed by a human chorus of "Gross!").

If an animal is not spayed or neutered, marking for a male is a way of letting females know that he is ready for a date! Spaying/neutering will sometimes see this subside, but there is still training involved.

Emotional Peeing

If other reasons are not present (territorial marking, submission, excitement, and/or pain), generally, peeing could be a training malfunction or a particularly strong emotion. If it is training, it is worth taking the time and starting over with a trainer. Tapping would help, but training would help more. There are always diapers, belly bands, and pee pads for dogs. Sadly, cats will end up in the shelter.

If it is emotionally based, there is a lot that can be done here. In Chinese medicine, the bladder and its sister meridian, the kidney, are associated with fear. As with territorial peeing, fear may be the underlying cause, whether it is due to change, loss of someone in the household (include grief in the script), and any other big change that could shift an animal's world.

In my years as an animal communicator, I have found worry to be an underlying emotion that accompanies peeing. With big change, often the household shifts a bit, and the animal may feel displaced or threatened as to their position in their everyday domestic life.

There may also be conflict with other animals in the household, which would lead to anxiety and frustration.

Physical Causes for Peeing

Humans often jump to the conclusion that inappropriate peeing has behavioral causes. The truth is that much of it is not, and sadly, many animals end up not only in the shelter but euthanized because they are misdiagnosed. One of the worst reasons for inappropriate peeing in cats is as the aftermath of declawing. The act of declawing is actually an amputation of the tops of what would be their fingers.

Urinary Tract Infections (UTI's) are a leading cause for inappropriate peeing, as is kidney and/or bladder disease. These are easily diagnosed, but two conditions that are exceptionally painful and don't get diagnosed easily are idiopathic cystitis (which can lead to crystals and a clogging of the urethra that could result in a major surgery, if not death) and osteoarthritis/joint pain.

Idiopathic cystitis may be accompanied by other bigger diseases or conditions, such as diabetes or Cushing's disease, but it is its own pretty terrible experience. It is a swelling of the bladder wall or urethra. If it goes undiagnosed for a long time, it leads to a thickening of the bladder wall. Any sort of pressure emotionally would feel like pressure physically, and the bladder would fill swiftly with no room to store it, so that the pee comes out rapidly, wherever they are, whenever they are feeling that tension. Having done animal medical intuition on thousands of animals with this condition, it is very painful and comes on quickly, feeling like an ongoing emergency in the body. Sadly, this gets overlooked until it is a medical emergency.

Osteoarthritis is very probable in 90 percent of all older animals over the age of 12. Because people don't see an animal limping, they don't understand that the hind end ain't what it used to be. Much of the breakdown in an animal that is older is bilateral, so they aren't going to look completely lame. With a discerning eye, you will see a little hitch in the giddy-up.

Unless an animal is a complainer (which most cats are not) or there is a lot of licking on a paw to indicate some pain or tissue damage, you might never know. Animals are stoic. They must be. Unless you are the apex predator, you are predator or prey. Dogs and cats in their wildest form are predators until they get old, and then, like the rest of us, they are prey. So they don't complain.

Overstimulation

Never underestimate overstimulation. If an animal is "excitement-peeing," it is just that: The animal is excited and can't control itself. Usually, they outgrow this, but not overnight.

Submissive peeing is a little harder. It is usually fear-based and may involve a bad memory of being in big trouble for something.

Let's Break It Down

No matter the outcome on this discovery as to why the animal is engaging in these behaviors, usually, it is suffering as it is unable to communicate exactly what is going on. It is nothing less than frustration and/or heartbreak for the human.

Many people like to dismiss inappropriate peeing as the animal just being pissed off, but there are many deeper emotions that might be contributing, so avoid making a quick diagnosis. While the animal may, in fact, be pissed off, there are a lot of other feelings attending the party, such as grief, fear, worry, anxiety, feeling threatened, and frustration. And for the human, the feelings could range from being angry, frustrated, heartbroken, confused, and feeling like a failure.

With the excitement peeing of a puppy, that could be a quick round of tapping a few times a day with a script that begins with "I'm so excited, OMG, I'm so excited!" and ends in a perfect world with "I'm all grown up and can control myself. I'm a big girl/boy now."

Commitment to Harmony

After discovering that one of my own cats had cystitis, I worked with holistic veterinarian Dr. Jill Todd for acupuncture and cold laser treatments. I created an anti-inflammatory diet/supplementation regime and tapped with my cat. He had been the one to pick out Delilah, when she was a puppy, as the next new member of the household, but the whirlwind energy of a puppy turned out to be a lot for my two-year-old cat Henry, who wasn't entirely sure of his place now.

After tapping a lot on worry, I always ended the session with statements about how he was the heart of the household and that everything emotional would be synthesized through him. It wasn't until the tapping that I realized how significant his role was. Since then, we have had no issues. In knowing who he was through this deep work, I personally made a vow to always allow for harmony to be the status of the household; in this way, everyone was free to process their emotions but we were all a bigger unit. I became the "emotional leader" of our collective. I talk about emotional leadership in both of my previous books, but the importance of it gets accentuated through this work.

Other Unwanted Behaviors

As a small dog with a big personality, Finn took it upon himself to alert the neighbors by barking loudly at them when they were in their own backyard—apparently, this was not a big hit with the neighbors. Finn was the third dog adopted into a pack of four dogs, two adults (Janet and Dave), and their two boisterous sons.

Great attempts were made to keep Finn in, but he took his self-imposed job quite seriously and could jet out the door and run up the hill to bark in seconds. To make matters worse, Janet has some physical limitations, so she couldn't crawl up the hill to catch Finn in action.

Dave hit the wall with the situation after they received a warning from animal control and was ready to find another home for Finn. This devastated Janet, and she even witnessed a tear coming out of Finn's eye.

Janet called me for an animal communication session, where I discovered that Finn was wired to be on high alert and still embedding himself in this family, with its mildly chaotic home life, bouncy kids, two high-powered working adults, and neighbors who dared to go in their own backyard.

In a household like Janet and Dave's, a lot is going on all the time: homework and activities for the kids, work deadlines, and household stresses for the adults. And where does Finn fit in with the other dogs?

EFT was helpful for both the human and the dog. We tapped on Finn to help him feel safe, and tapped on Janet's sadness about Dave demanding they get rid of the dog and her anxiety about her perception of Finn's naughty behavior.

I am happy to say that Finn is still with his family. He calmed down about his place in the household, and Janet is more aware of her feelings about his behavior. The household is bouncier than ever, but Finn is very happy.

Separation Anxiety

Separation happens very early for animals, even before they are weaned, and from then on, they must get used to a series of separations. As discussed in Chapter 5, animals experience grief often, beginning with those earliest years, and in some, it compounds and leads to deep-seated feelings.

Some animals don't feel safe during that constant separating process. They have never learned to self-soothe, have had little to no training, and/or suffer from low self-esteem. When it comes to separation anxiety, you need all hands on deck to head it off, because as they get older or the longer this behavior is entrenched in their being, the harder it is to train/heal out of them—not impossible but definitely a challenge.

Long term, because the animal is in fight-or-flight state so often, it takes a toll on their adrenal glands and their nervous and immune systems. To help reverse or at least manage the behavior and the subsequent damage it can produce, it may require a veterinarian, a trainer, an EFT practitioner, and maybe even a behaviorist. It requires treating it from every angle, from calming foods to new behaviors.

Some animals are completely unglued if their person leaves the room—they panic. Birds that were captive-born have imprinted onto humans because they never met their mother and depend on them. We see separation anxiety mostly in dogs, but dogs that are overly connected to the other dog(s) in the household can experience separation anxiety from leaving each other. And of course, horses can be very herd-bound. If one herd member takes a step in a different direction, there is a rallying cry for the horse to come right back.

Sometimes, separation anxiety looks destructive. It is important to understand if your animal is simply bored and destructive or if it is truly anxious. Those would be two very different tapping scripts! One would be "I'm bored, I'm bored, why not eat the couch?" The other would be based on earlier experiences, such as being afraid of being alone or being sad that everyone is gone, then working through the panic. The script would end with a lot about the animal being confident, being okay in their own body, being able to feel safe and knowing all is well in the world.

Tapping on the human as well as the animal is vital to success. Often the human feels responsible, guilty, frustrated, and helpless.

Those are some of the big feelings that usually come out of the human investigation.

Performance Blocks

I use the word "performance" for working animals, as well as animals that are showing or in any sort of competitive event. Performance can be the display or presentation of something, as in a performance in the theater or a concert. For animals this may be entertainment, but more often, this sort of performance is a competitive event.

Performance can also be the process or action of carrying out a certain task or action. This would be more like service animals, such as horses in therapeutic riding centers or guide dogs.

In any case, the function that is expected to be performed carries an expectation on behalf of the human and the animal, and this can create a certain pressure. Like people, some animals enjoy that pressure.

Performance Blocks in Service Animals

People who don't really know animals say that animals don't pick their jobs, but if you know animals, much of the time they have, in fact, picked their perfect scenario. I have met hundreds if not thousands of failed service animals that are frolicking in people's backyards and enjoying being on their portion of the human bed.

That said, I have met equally as many service animals that LOVE their job and relish their ability to do it perfectly. Going back to the concept of pressure, not only is this type of work perfect for an animal but these are the types of animals that add pressure to themselves!

"Perfect" is the operative word there. More times than not, a service animal has a Type A personality, so if their service isn't perfect, they can shut down or act out. Between the guide dog world, emotional support animals, and therapeutic riding centers, many people and centers have hired me as an animal communicator for the last 30 years, and most of them have benefited from EFT.

No matter what species or what job, if one thing goes wrong, the sense of failure and impending doom for the animal is palpable. They have a true sense of life or death for the human. When I have tapped with animals in therapeutic riding centers and/or guide dogs, the sense of responsibility for the human(s) is almost overwhelming. If a horse or dog has failed in this duty, it feels it deeply, and may feel sadness, overwhelm, frustration, and confusion. For the human, whether it is the guardian, physical therapist, or person who needs the guide dog, they often feel sad, let down, helpless, frustrated, and confused.

In cases where an animal has to be retired as the result of a breakdown in behavior or the physical body, both parties may feel a lot of grief. It is the end of a working relationship, a career, a service, and most importantly, a deep friendship.

Buster the Emotional Sponge

Buster is a horse who took on everything for everyone. If his quadriplegic person was having a bad period at school at 3 p.m. on Monday and Wednesday and his epileptic person was having more episodes on Tuesday and Thursday, he was feeling it—not only was he feeling it but he was also so empathic, he was taking it on.

We tapped on his sorrow, sadness, and deep, deep feeling of being out of control. At the end of the tapping, we envisioned him as a safe island for so many that he couldn't take on their pain; he could only be their safe island. This was profound for Buster and his future. He had a renewed start with all of the people depending on him after this refresher using animal communication and tapping.

Because Buster had many humans looking after him, the main physical therapist, Jodi, was the one who involved me and called the board of directors to get my help. In the end, Jodi was also the one we tapped with. We tapped on her guilt of not realizing how taxed he was and her helplessness when he seemed to be losing it.

In the end, Buster went to work that next week with a renewed sense of his work. Jodi made sure that everyone around him was aware of when he was overworked. Last I heard, they were all in stride and of service with the workload of helping challenged humans.

Performance Blocks in Competitive Events

Over the years, I have connected with thousands of animals that compete in some form or fashion. As a young girl, I rode Western competitively with my horse through seventh grade, but after I got an English saddle for Christmas at the age of 13, there was no turning back. Middle school through college, I competed mostly in show jumping and what was then referred to as "English Equitation," which is judged on how well the rider can handle the horse and their balance. Now I prefer dressage but don't compete.

In a heartbeat, I can flash back to being "in the zone" with Honeyhorse, my horse, racing bareback over trails at what seemed like 40 mph, with the pattern of the trail memorized of when to duck a branch or lean forward to jump a log lying across the path, and then next day, dressed formally, competing at a horseshow. These are some of my favorite childhood memories, and because of them, I have re-created being in that zone with all my animals in some form or fashion, particularly my horses.

I have always been able to relate to people and animals that compete, but whether you win or lose a competition or are out in the field walking your horse or dog, on the couch with your cat, or attending a big event with your animal, being "in the zone" is the space that everyone yearns to attain.

Honeyhorse and I had plenty of times when it was the opposite of being "in the zone" for us, and I know what this feels like. From perfecting the "bite" moment in Schutzhund, a type of competition for dogs that involves tracking, obedience, and protection; to creating a bolder jump for the next horse show; to getting the final obedience title because the dog finally followed the scent; to being calm enough and in the moment enough to pick up the right lead canter; to finally sorting out the weave polls—I have used animal communication and animal medical intuition with many human/animal competitive teams to break apart those moments when "the zone" slipped away so that they could get that back.

Regardless of it being a physical, mental, emotional, and/or relationship issue, EFT has been extraordinary in bringing clarity on how to stay in the moment, almost like a GPS, to guide both partners back to "the zone," where it all flows and possibility is in the air.

For the most part, the higher the competition, the more the team is used to living largely "in the zone," so the more is at stake. Many unnatural things go on at an event, no matter what species or type of event. While training for a competition at home, nobody can anticipate the challenges—large indoor arenas with sharp barking bouncing off high ceilings; the smell of human foods alongside urine and poop; so many people; so many animals, including animals in heat (exciting!); the audience clapping after an event; bright floodlights in the evening; and so much more. That makes "the zone" so much more prized, as it is a safety net for any animal in these unnatural circumstances.

At the end of the day, the connection is usually dropped as a result of the human's nerves. Of course, there are occasions when the animal gets distracted or spooks, but the moment can be saved if the human is super solid and committed to "the zone." Tapping on the human becomes as important as tapping on the horse for whatever fears, phobias, or awarenesses the animal has.

NOTE: For a sample tapping session template, please refer to Let's Tap in Chapter 5 and the Appendix.

Juniper

I met a horse named Juniper at an international horse show, where he was being shown by his trainer Melody. Juniper had come from a prestigious show barn in Europe. His show record as a dressage horse was well worth the price of admission, meaning that someone had paid a lot of money for him and had hired Melody to show him at a high level, as had happened in Europe.

Only now, he was shutting down in the show ring on the international circuit, and no amount of money was worth it for his trainer to face that humiliation.

He was magnificent at home—humble, sensitive, giving, and athletic.

Sadly, all of those wonderful descriptions of his true essence are what got him where he was, and he was pushed very hard at a barn in Europe because of those qualities. Juniper was a superstar at home when he was ridden, but in the show ring, the pressure to perform was just too great.

When I communicated with Juniper, I got that sense of him and what had happened in the show ring. Being sensitive and experiencing that much pressure, he just went inside himself. He "disappeared" for the rider and, in turn, felt like Melody "disappeared" for him, so that when he was looking for somewhere safe, she was gone.

When I described all of that to Melody, she described him as the most willing and giving horse she's ever known, saying: "That is exactly what happens at home. So, every time I take him to a show, I think, *This will be different. Someone, someone will finally see who he is.*"

His person felt exactly the same way. Both the trainer and Juniper's person were so sad. They had invested heavily in a famous Olympian for coaching, and it wasn't just the financial investment—both his person and trainer were in love with him.

I offered tapping, and because they had seen positive results from other horses I have worked with over the years, they were up for it.

I asked Melody what it was like to have him "disappear" under her. Was there another experience where she had had to cope but had zero control? She thought for a moment and then, with tears in her eyes, shared a story about her dad dying while she was in high school.

I tapped on her first, and we had a very emotional tapping session, even though the loss of her dad had taken place 20 years ago. Then we tapped on the feeling of being out of control with Juniper, because he was just gone and is giant in size. That alone can be scary, and the feeling of being suddenly out of control was just like when her father died.

For Juniper, we tapped on his big sensitivity, the sadness of being pushed and not seen, the harsh pressure of that dressage world in Europe, and the ultimate shutdown, where he went inside himself because nothing was safe.

We turned it into a perfect world, where Melody had his back. Melody was taking care of him. They could do it together. We had a beautiful visualization as the ending of the tapping.

Juniper got his highest score in the US competition that weekend and qualified for more events. He and Melody had a flawless ride. It was gorgeous, and I was able to see it.

I believe that he was retired from the show ring relatively soon after the tapping. His person didn't want to put that kind of pressure on any horse. I later discovered that there was a class action suit against the European trainer for this very abuse: breaking down so many horses of this sensitive nature.

Magic

Magic was the opposite of Juniper: He didn't shut down when things were distracting; instead, he had a tendency to bolt. Magic was the epitome of a stunning, solid-muscle horse with a dazzling personality. He inspired many with his athleticism and charm. Everybody loved Magic. Especially his person, Jennie Hlavacek.

Magic loved EFT. He would not only get relaxed from tapping; he would go to sleep! That relaxed all the humans, too. Jennie knew that the more relaxed the animal, the better he will perform.

I flew several times to be with them and tap on Magic before his big classes at the horse shows. If I couldn't be there in person, I was a phone call away. I woke up in the middle of the night to tap on him remotely in Europe a few times. After each tapping, he entered the arena with his elegant rider and got to be the Zen horse we all knew him to be at home. We tapped on containing his energy within his four legs and completely trusting his rider.

The night classes with the floodlights and the people were hardest for him, especially in the showgrounds in Del Mar in Southern California. The horse would go down a ramp in the dark and enter a super-bright arena with grandstands full of people. One time when I couldn't fly down to be with them because I was teaching EFT, the whole class got to witness me leading the tapping with Magic while on the phone with Jennie, the rider, while her friend did the tapping in the stall.

7

Relationships and Dynamics

I imagine that there are many of us who see a picture of a sad-looking dog on the internet and know that we could spend the rest of our life with that beloved. We know in our heart, when we look in those eyes through the interwebs, that that is our dog/cat/horse/bird. The next thing we know, we have arranged a veterinarian, whatever paperwork is necessary, a flight, and that's it—we have moved our new animal soul mate in.

Yet, if that were a human on a dating site and those same sad eyes called out to you, would you plan to have a lifelong committed partnership with that person? Er, no. You would quickly scroll on by.

Soul mates come in all forms, including animal companions. When we look at our lifelong relationships with beings, often we are closest to the animals in our lives. Many husbands of equestrians know that their marriage works because their wife has a beautiful, devoted horse. With animals, we don't rely on language in the same way we do with humans; there is a mutual depth and wisdom that goes far beyond words into a communication that is far less sophisticated yet far more evolved. We enter a connection, a communion, a place where we don't need words—a space where the souls connect.

Our households may also be a container for animals that are soul mates or forever devoted to each other. Often, a devoted companion animal will die soon after the first one died. Just as with humans, heartbreak is real for animals in their relationships with each other. We have a paradoxical history with animals, a slow flirt from wolves and lions living in caves with humans, to humans worshipping cats in Egypt, to horses living in tents with humans and evolving to the equines and bovines helping us build civilization, to dogs helping to be companions and guidance for everything from PTSD to the blind, and so much more.

All the while, torture in the name of science, sacrifice in the name of religion/culture, objectification in the name of entertainment, and pleasure from killing in the name of sport can come from the same human that is capable of a soul mate relationship beyond words with their beloved dog.

We are witnessing the potential extinction of wildlife, all in the name of human greed. Those same dog lovers will wear makeup that was tested on a dog that didn't have a soul mate but lost an eye for them. And millions of not-so-lucky animals are dying a loveless death in a shelter genocide in the name of irresponsibility.

Yet, as an animal communicator/energy healer for animals for over 30 years, I continue to see (and experience) relationships that have no words big enough to contain the amount of love and devotion from both parties.

It is proven that the experience of love, safety, and affection from animals releases oxytocin, the bonding hormone in humans that also reduces stress. It has been found that dogs also release oxytocin when they are in an engaging, loving, safe relationship with humans. It is only proven in dogs, but we can only imagine, when we see the cross-species relationships that are so delicious, that this oxytocin must be released in other animals, too. I feel that same love chemical when I say good morning to the ravens nesting high above my hay shed when I feed my horses their breakfast. I pretend that the ravens feel the same way.

Caroline Myss, *New York Times* bestselling author on subjects from mysticism to wellness, says that your soul mate is not that romantic fantasy; rather, it is the one who stretches us. Sometimes, we get stretched beyond our wildest dreams—by the one who isn't perfect, the one who isn't who we pictured going into old age with, the one who didn't train easily, the one who was a little off in the distance while the rest of the dogs or cats played.

Those are the ones who stretch us and make us better humans. Those are the ones who are as much our soul mate as that easy-breezy first dog/horse/cat we had as a child that we romanticize, compare every animal to, and measure ourselves by. That isn't fair to the memory of that perfect animal, to us, and especially not fair to the animal in front of us. I have been guilty of the comparison myself.

When I've been tapping with people, in the investigation phase, I hear things like:

- "All of my friends have the perfect spouse, the perfect job, the perfect car, and the perfect pet. And my cat, well, . . . "

- "Everyone else has a dog that doesn't growl at the neighbor like mine does." (In their mind, the entire neighborhood has made their dog out to be the antichrist.)
- "All my friends have cats that seem to make it to the litter box.
- "I can't sleep all night without fearing a fight will break out among their animals."
- "I've had dogs my whole life, but this one . . . "
- "Why can't they just get along?"
- "I am a hostage to my animals."

As you are creating your investigation for yourself, it is important to give expression to this inside voice. These are the sorts of feelings that are deeply harbored and have as much to do with the distance in the relationship as anything. Allowing this to come up and be expressed is what is going to enhance the relationship.

Just for the record, I have had several equine, canine, and feline soul mates (the good news about animal soul mates is that we don't have to be monogamous). Each of those relationships required a certain amount of mutual work, dedication, and willingness to work together to make it great.

Lucca: All You Need Is Love, Right?

Lucca not only barked at anything and everything that came into his household but would also be rattled by the experience for days.

Lucca is a 10-year-old, gorgeous (supermodel) cocker spaniel who was adopted by Maria and her husband when he was about five years old. He had come from a hoarding case, where animals were packed into a space that was unsanitary. That is all he had known—there were his family.

Maria had fostered and rescued many cocker spaniels before Lucca, and love was the elixir that had shifted everyone so far. Not Lucca. He stayed in this skittish space, and it was a good year before her husband Steven was able to even touch Lucca.

Through animal communication and EFT, Maria discovered a lot about her own feelings as she walked through the process. Prior to EFT, she had pigeonholed Lucca as being a "problem child" and couldn't fathom that he had a playful heart. She felt that it was her job to help him not freak out, and he obliged because he is a pleaser. Maria felt it was a deficit in her that he wasn't better. In some ways, she felt sorry for him, so he was never able to rise to the occasion.

Now, she appreciates him a lot more. He follows her everywhere, as though he is her witness. He is more in love with her than her husband is, and she certainly welcomes that devotion. He's more playful, and in turn, Maria is more playful with him. She isn't embarrassed by the loud barking, and she doesn't feel as guilty anymore. Lucca still barks a bit, but it is more hollow and not as apocalyptic. He also recovers immediately. It isn't a three-day event if someone comes to the house to look at the washing machine.

After training as an animal communicator and energy healer herself now, Maria will have more compassion than ever for the human going through this disappointment and self-blame, as well as help elevate the status of the animal.

Love is the answer, as well as a few other things. I always say that the four big tools to shift a behavior, relationship, or household dynamics are:

- Animal Communication
- Energy Healing
- Training
- Management

I put *animal communication* first, because when any being is heard or seen, the healing begins and then, when you bring in *energy healing,* you can help the trauma release. With *training,* you have the opportunity to redirect the energy that was going elsewhere. You are creating new neuropathways.

When none of the first three things work the way you want them to, there is always *management,* but often, management is where the feelings of love for the animal start to break down. Feelings of resentment, frustration, and often shame are associated with management and can make the relationship more complex.

A lot of trainers will talk about how you can love an animal to death. You can love them so much and believe they need total freedom and zero boundaries that you then watch the animal run into the street. Holistic veterinarians will talk about how you can love an animal so much you give them too many treats and send their system into a metabolic disorder.

Boundaries are essential in order for a shift to be able to take place. This is sometimes called "tough love." The more animals you have, the quicker you watch it cascade into chaos if you aren't on top of exactly who is doing what, who likes who, and who is ready to pounce on who.

A best-case scenario, in which everyone in a relationship shows their best self, is what makes the world go around. In the worst possible scenario, it is what keeps the world at war and division among humans at an epic level. Placing our attention on the smallest relationships and watching the love is like a petri dish for the world. Finding ways to restore balance and harmony within our households will ripple out as a force-field for good.

Animal and Human Relationship Blocks

Working as an animal communicator and energy healer, I had a work week for many years that was broken up into maybe two days of me driving from client to client and meeting the animal(s) in person, and then doing back-to-back sessions by phone and meeting the animal(s) and their human(s) remotely the rest of the week. As I did my work, my title could have been Animal/Human Relationship Specialist.

If it was a family dynamic, I would listen to each animal. One dog might believe they were higher in the hierarchy, but then, I would listen to the new dog, which saw that the systems in the household were falling apart and someone had to take over. And then with complete neutrality, I would hear the humans. It always felt like once all of it was on the table, it was so clear, and it came back together quite naturally, and if not, an EFT session completed it.

I think that one key part of the EFT session is that when you must look at yourself in the investigation process, you already start to shift. When you are tapping on behalf of your animal, it is like a mini animal communication session and your perception of the animal will shift.

Relationships are everything. Because there are so many animals dumped in shelters or returned to small rescues after years of living in a home, I try to understand the commitment level of the human before I invest my heart 100 percent. I would rather hear "I'm not sure if this dog really fits our household" than "Oh, we will do anything for her" and then, two weeks later, find out they returned her to the rescue after four years in their home.

In other words, I like to know what somebody's "family values" are. One little behavioral issue can start fraying the fabric of the relationship, like a crafty moth, and then the structure will fall away unless the love and commitment are there.

Afton Hughes, one of the animal communication teachers of CWALU, had been a dog trainer before becoming an animal communicator/energy healer, and she has also been in the rescue world forever, as well as running some nonprofits. To say she is an animal professional is an understatement. While Afton was in the CWALU program and learning energy healing and everything else, we had the opportunity to work on her dog Leila. When Leila came back to live with Afton after nine years and started biting her other pack members, you can imagine how Afton was feeling when she couldn't see it coming.

Afton loved Leila and picked her out of a shelter to foster her. Leila was submissive and fearful, but Afton trusted her, and her own mother fell in love with her and kept her. Afton's mother went through several life changes (a divorce after a 25-year marriage and then a new marriage), plus, she was clinically depressed. When Afton's mother decided to travel the world without the dog, nobody was more surprised than Afton, except for maybe Leila.

It was not just a "back off" bite from Leila during weekly trips to the vet so the other dogs could get stitches, painkillers, or antibiotics that left Afton upset. She was mad at Leila and frustrated with her own inability to manage it. Ultimately, she wanted Leila gone, as her own dogs weren't safe.

Afton said: "I felt sorry for her because I couldn't understand her. I had exhausted the things that would have triggered it. Everything is very structured."

This was not a warm fuzzy household for a grieving dog like Leila. After tapping in class, the incidents with Leila went way down, and the situation is now managed. Afton can clearly see the signs of when Leila is agitated and can get her her own space for a while. Leila chooses to be with the rest of the family in harmony now.

Bison!

Glasses clinking, a tennis shoe skidding making the sound of rubber meeting a gymnasium floor, a timer in the kitchen and God forbid, a fire alarm can send Bison, an 11-year-old Lab/Great Dane mix into an escapade of barking incessantly while staring at the ceiling.

Linda could clap or use her voice loudly to stop it, but the reverberation of the disturbance leaves the other two dogs—Chaka, an eight-year-old pit bull mix, and Lefty, a two-year-old pit bull—completely unnerved. Not to mention it sends her husband Keith over the edge.

The move from Seattle to Arizona didn't help this any. In fact, it escalated. Linda joined CWALU and was able to tap with one of the teachers, Kaki Decker, and after only one session, things changed. Linda feels as though Bison now thinks about it when she hears a sound. She looks around and checks in with herself. Kaki also tapped with Linda, and Linda is no longer anticipating the disruption and feels closer to Bison.

Breaking Down Human to Animal Relationships

Once you have a clear understanding, whether it be from an animal communication session or just a hunch as to what your animal is thinking/feeling about their habits, you can start to break it down for yourself.

The more honest you are about how you and others are feeling, the easier it will be to remove the wedge that the behavior and those feelings are creating, so that you are coming from a space of compassion and possibility. Our animals always respond to that.

Animal to Animal Relationship

I find the depth of the relationships that each of my animals has with each other fascinating. Years ago, I had a Black Lab named Isabella. She would talk my cat Henry into shoving everything off the counter so they could share whatever food was there. My horse Anya takes care of my older horse, Gabrielle. Buster Keaton the cat grooms each of the dogs before our morning meditation. The ravens clean up the food bowls and surrounding areas after my horses have had breakfast. Okay, the raven isn't one of my animals, but her nest is on the property, and

I feel like we are cousins at the very least. She walks around, a lot and doesn't bother flying off when I come near!

Anya and Drakkar

Right before the COVID pandemic in early 2020, Drakkar came into my life and joined the herd. Eight-year-old Drakkar is a 17-hand (that means big) thoroughbred, and he is so cute. Every morning, when I go out to feed the animals, I look at him and think, *My God, I live with the Brad Pitt of horses!*

Anya is my gorgeous Hungarian Warmblood, a dream riding horse, but to say that she did not like Drakkar is an understatement. Between her and my elder horse Gabrielle, their squeals made a cat hissing seem like nothing.

Anya's prior home was a prestigious dressage barn, where she had not lived as part of a herd. When she came to me in 2012, I put her out with Gabrielle and Rollie, a tall, dark, and handsome thoroughbred. At first, Anya didn't want anything to do with the other horses, but in no time, she had her own herd.

When Rollie died, the collective grief that I, Anya, and Gabrielle felt, a fog of Pacific Northwest tears and rain, was enough to send us out of the Seattle area and into the sunshine of California. Now, here we were. I had never had a herd challenge and didn't know what to do about Anya and Drakkar's dislike of one another.

One night, I was driving home from dinner, contemplating how I was going to get these horses to get along, when a song I always associate with Rollie came on the radio. In an instant, I knew that Anya was still really grieving Rollie. At this point, Rollie had been gone for five years, but he was the first horse to accept Anya in a herd, and who was I to judge the extended grief?

The next morning, over breakfast, I tapped on "This is no Rollie. Who does this guy think he is? I'm still grieving" and kept it going on the grieving theme until I felt Anya release. Then I moved the tapping to "Drakkar is kind of cute."

After the tapping, I let Drakkar out, and he came over to Anya's stall in a hopeful truce. The two horses sniffed each other's noses over the fence, and she instantly went into heat. That was it, they've been in love ever since. I often tell them now to get a stall—too much public display of affection!

Honey Bear and Menorah

To watch Menorah saunter across the barnyard is like watching a movie star on the red carpet. She is honestly, the most breathtakingly beautiful exotic pig I've ever seen. From her distinctive ears, which she tosses around like someone flipping their hair, to her eyes, which look like she is wearing eyeliner, to the swing of her hind end with each sexy step, Menorah has got it going on.

Menorah was meant to be someone's Christmas dinner, but when she gave birth to eight piglets, somehow the human family didn't feel like they could eat her and contacted The Gentle Barn.

The Gentle Barn rescues farm animals and helps heal them. In return, those animals give back to humans by serving as ambassadors for their species and helping special groups, such as kids at risk, veterans, and more, who visit on Sundays. Often, humans that have been abused or tossed out see themselves in the beautiful animals at The Gentle Barn, and there is nothing more healing than being seen or heard.

When The Gentle Barn founders Ellie Laks and Jay Weiner heard about this sow and her babies, they drove up from Santa Clarita to Oregon on Christmas Day to pick up the beautiful family. Their plan was that Menorah and her babies would fit right in with the other pigs, goats, sheep, chickens, llamas, and emu Earl. One of the animals, Honey Bear, a giant pig, was genetically modified for consumption, hence his size, and it was hoped that not only would they accept one another but also have a sweet family. Neither Honey Bear nor Menorah were having any of *that*! In fact, hostilities broke out between them almost immediately. Menorah may have taken the first reactive step, but Honey Bear was soon on the defense.

From then on, to keep the peace, barnyard hours had to be split between Honey Bear being out when Menorah was in a stall with her eight growing piglets, then the two switching. This is not ideal in summer, as Santa Clarita is in northwest Los Angeles County, an inland high desert location, and no matter how many fans are blowing on animals in the stall, being in a 12-by-12 space during the day is hot.

Ellie had me out to communicate with the pigs. First, I communicated with Honey Bear, and he shared that he had been beaten up by other pigs in the past and was pretty defensive and wasn't having any of that. Zeus, the other large pig hero of The Gentle Barn, had recently passed, and they too had had to be kept separate because of occasional aggression.

In our communication, Menorah shared with me that she viewed all male pigs as rapists, based on her previous experiences with them, and that this was her second time being a mom. While she's a great mom, she didn't like the way she was treated by the male pigs.

The next time I came over to The Gentle Barn, we were going to do the EFT tapping and then put all the pigs together to see if it worked. The staff had large pig boards ready to go in case it was a repeat of the first meeting.

I tapped on Honey Bear first. We tapped on how bullied he'd been and how tough he had had to be, but deep down he was a softie and Menorah would be safe with him. At the end, we did a little visualization of the big family of pigs in the barnyard.

With Menorah, we tapped on the rape culture of male pigs, and how out of control it always is and ended with "Honey Bear is safe." At the end, I did the same visualization with her that I had done with Honey Bear, that of a big, happy, pig family.

When it came time to put them together, while Ellie was reluctant, her husband Jay and the staff were ready. If it didn't work, it didn't work.

The stall doors were opened, and some of the babies spilled out into the yard. Both Honey Bear and Menorah entered the barnyard at about the same time.

They went their separate ways at first but were very curious about each other. There was peace in the air. They started getting closer and closer, and eventually, they were hanging out.

Honey Bear has now passed, but since that day, he and Menorah acted like husband and wife. Menorah would tuck her babies into the family stall and then tuck herself into a night with her man, Honey Bear.

Breaking Down Animal to Animal Relationships

Once you have a clear understanding, whether it be from an animal communication session or just a hunch as to what your animals are thinking/feeling about their relationship with each other, you can start to break it down and put together the big feelings of each (or all) of them into a script.

Sometimes, as in the case of Menorah and Honey Bear, Ellie and the staff hardly knew Menorah, and we could have tapped on Ellie about her apprehension of putting them together. But if it is a situation you have been living with for a while, it is probable that you have big feelings. Again, the more honest you are with yourself, the less your feelings/projections will be compounding the situation.

NOTE: For a sample tapping session template, please refer to Let's Tap in Chapter 5 and the Appendix.

8

Wellness

Many energy-healing techniques involve having the animal relax in order to engage the parasympathetic nervous system. The autonomic nervous system controls most of the bodily functions we don't have to think about: heart, digestion, circulation, the endocrine and reproduction systems, and more.

The sympathetic nervous system is about fight or flight, while the parasympathetic nervous system is about rest and digest, the restful state that is necessary for healing and restoration.

The beauty of EFT is that we are setting things up to flourish. Tapping not only engages the parasympathetic nervous system but also allows the body to reach homeostasis. *Homeostasis* refers to dynamic equilibrium in the body whereby, both chemically and physically, our whole system is stabilized, even if things are challenging it. Think of it as being like a body thermostat—our bodies love to be in this state.

Whether our animal companion has an illness, an injury, a surgery, or had a rough start requiring lots of antibiotics and now has a funky tummy, a systemic condition, or the like—all of these challenges can put them in survival mode, a mild fight-or-flight state, whereby they are just getting by and not thriving. This doesn't necessarily help or hurt their situation; however, it means that it can take longer to reach a desired outcome.

EFT finds the emotional block or the underlying emotional cause to a physical condition, and that helps dissolve the block or give light to its origins and provides the homeostasis and ability to thrive in one shot!

Often, as guardians, we are not sure what to do, because our animal's well-being is linked to our own well-being, and therefore, our own stress level. As much as we want to immediately use EFT on our animals to tap out the illness or lameness, we would do well to tap on ourselves first. Often our own stress or worry can be contributing to feelings of survival rather than flourishing.

In her dog Boogie's final years, my friend Erica often tapped on herself because she didn't want to make a wrong decision. Boogie had so many complications in his elder years that one decision could help him bounce back, while another decision could be a gateway to another crisis. She tapped on her fear of making a wrong decision. It worked for her, as she made excellent decisions until his very last breath.

A health challenge can make us question everything we know, so tapping can be a powerful tool in the way that Erica used it. As noted earlier, we can also find "secondary gains" as to why our animal might remain lame or sick when it is not life-threatening. Are we spending more time with them? Do they get more love?

The other day, my dogs were racing up the hill from the horses to get their own breakfast, and my dog Penelope, a two-year-old flying Muppet (there's Border Collie in there, maybe Italian greyhound, and Kelpie), ran into a pole with her right hip and cried and crumpled.

I went running over and examined her leg and hip. I discovered that there were no broken bones, no swelling, no pain to the touch, and probably just a hip and ego bruise, and since she is the only dog in my household small enough to sit on my lap, I held her there while I did energy work on her hip.

After I removed my hands, she shot off to finish the wild play with my other two dogs, but as she came bursting into the catio, where the dogs dine with the cats, she suddenly only had three working legs and hobbled around in my presence.

I went into the kitchen and peered out at her in the catio, where she was now using all four legs fine. Then, when I came back out, she was suddenly three-legged lame again.

Need a little attention?

Pain

According to online encyclopedia *Wikipedia*, pain is:

- a distressing feeling often caused by intense or damaging stimuli. The International Association for the Study of Pain defines pain as "an unpleasant sensory and emotional experience associated with, or resembling that associated with, actual or potential tissue damage." In medical diagnosis, pain is regarded as a symptom of an underlying condition.

Pain can create long-term stress and just plain old not thinking right. It can bring about a lot of behavioral challenges, as discussed in Chapter 6. It can dim the life force. Using EFT for pain can help someone start to think about and experience something else. Again, if you are feeling sorry or guilty for your animal's condition, using EFT to release those feelings creates a lighter space for the animal to heal.

Lameness

Susie and her granddaughter Carly share a love of horses, and Carly stables her eight-year-old horse Baby, a cute, off-the-track thoroughbred and life partner, at Susie's house. Baby's name fits his personality—a little too curious, full of beans, but as in love with Carly as she is with him.

One day, Baby got a puncture wound above the fetlock and tore the suspensory digital flexor tendon—in other words, in a complicated location and injuring a necessary tendon. Susie's local vet treated the injury loosely, since she couldn't stitch it because of the location, and put Baby on pain medication and antibiotics.

Baby was not getting better, so Susie and Carly loaded him up and took him to the university hospital, where the vet shamed Susie for not coming in sooner and Carly felt completely deflated. Part of the problem was that no matter what level of care you give a horse like Baby, if they are not good about stall rest—that is, they can't stay still—they will keep reinjuring themselves, or at the very least have a long, long road to recovery. This is the sort of thing that ages the best of us.

Back at home, Baby's condition did not get better, and it didn't feel as though he was going to heal. Baby, Susie, and Carly were all pretty heartbroken about the situation, and their belief in a miracle was gone. Thankfully, Susie was studying with me at CWALU, and her last class before graduating was Energy Healing for Animals, so we do a lot of EFT in there. We set up on Zoom, so that the class could see Susie, Carly and Baby, and Susie and Carly could see all of us. I did the lead with the script, Susie followed with the camera on Baby and repeated after me, tapping on the points on Baby, and Carly was there for moral support.

The big feelings I tapped on Baby were his disappointment, his sadness, his anxiety from being in a stall all day and that he hated to let Carly down. There were some secondary gains—he was getting extra lunch and being pampered—but in a perfect world, he would have a miraculous healing, he and Carly would go back to dressage and the trails, and he could be out in the pasture with his herd buddies.

Something shifted in the barn aisle, and Carly lit up. For her heart to be unbroken and unshattered lifted her, and it made all the difference. Susie felt like we gave Baby permission to get better and that gravity had lifted and said "Okay, you can fly." Baby is sound now on all four legs. They all believe they had a miracle.

It Reminds Me of . . .

Vixie Elizabeth is an adorable Corgi and the master of Jill Todd, DVM, my business partner in Jill and Joan Healing. In fact, let's just say, Vixie Elizabeth owns Jill. Jill also has another goddess dog, Olive, a Rhodesian Ridgeback.

One day, Jill left treats in the crates and didn't realize until she found Vixie Elizabeth injured that Olive had pounced and gotten the treats she had left. Jill then went out of town and got a call from her pet sitter that Vixie Elizabeth couldn't stand and that her hind limbs weren't working.

Jill is an amazing holistic veterinarian, and has 10 million tools, but she knows too much about these things and, in her terror and sadness, immediately went to the worst-case scenario in her mind: "She'll either need back surgery or a cart."

The next morning, Vixie Elizabeth stood up and moved a bit, and slowly but surely, through rehab, acupuncture, cold laser, and more, regained her mobility. During that time, we did some big tapping.

Jill revealed that she knew she was anxious and worried about the future. She can't stand feeling scared about the future. She also was watching every step that Vixie Elizabeth was taking. When we got to the "reminds me of" part of the script, Jill said, "It reminds me of Rafiki, and we had to put him to sleep." (Rafiki was a Rhodesian Ridgeback with a back injury years prior, and Jill was still devastated, disappointed, and overwhelmingly sad that this is what she does for a living and couldn't save him.) That was big.

In the perfect world of the script, Jill wanted full recovery through the rehabilitation work and that she, Vixie Elizabeth, Olive, and her boyfriend Rodney would all go back to normal activities. By releasing the old buried Rafiki story, this recovery started to happen a lot faster.

My Brief Year Having a Healing Center

About the time my first book came out, in 2007, I fulfilled what had been a dream for more than a decade—my own healing center. Whether living in Los Angeles, Denver, South Florida, or the Seattle area, I had always created a healing circle with holistic veterinarians, chiropractors, nutritionists, massage therapists, saddle fitters, farriers, and more, but had yet to find the right location for a physical space for healing.

Upon my divorce, I moved to Seattle to be with my dying father and created just that. In fact, that is how I met Jill Todd in the last story—I stalked her, as I needed a holistic veterinarian, and all the while, she was stalking me, as she needed an animal communicator!

What I discovered after a year of living my dream of over 10 years is that it was not my dream. My friend Ellie Laks of The Gentle Barn says she thinks that dream was just a place holder for the school, CWALU. I would have to agree. I couldn't see it in my mind's eye, so the healing center made sense.

I'm not sure why I thought then that starting a school would be easier than starting a healing center, but that would be another book. The truth is, the new book *Communication with all Life,* was coming out, I had a dying father, and I was in the midst of a divorce.

Four Healing Stories

The next four stories are of animals that came to the healing center. Two of the horses stayed with me, and a dog and cat came in for bi-weekly appointments. They all left with bigger healing than expected.

I had so much going on, I couldn't appreciate how truly amazing it was. I do remember my friend Shannon called from Florida one day and asked, "How's it going up there in your new place?"

Very nonchalantly I replied, "Not much. Just a few miracles—dogs walking out of here, horses not lame. You know, the usual."

It wasn't until she started laughing that I realized, *Wow, some amazing stuff is going on here!*

Troy and Navicular Disease

One of the first miracles we had at the healing center was Troy, a horse diagnosed with navicular disease, a progressive disease that causes lameness (limping). Troy had been lame on and off for years.

Upon Troy's arrival, his person, Ava said, "We've tried everything. I hope this works." For many people, it is hard to move past what the Western medicine label or belief system is for any disease or condition.

We made several changes. Against common wisdom for this condition, we took his shoes off to allow for his feet to grow a little more and have better circulation. We changed his diet to a non-inflammatory diet. I worked on his whole body and both of his front feet using scalar energy. I have healing machines that stimulate circulation and promote cellular healing, so we had all of that going on as well.

When I would do a medical intuition scan, I felt so confident that we had a miracle, yet when I would get him trotting circles in the round pen there was still this ever-so-slight lameness.

I remember walking back to the barn aisle with him and asking Ava, "What would it look like for this horse to be healed?"

Her blank stare said everything to me. I asked her some key questions and discovered that both she and Troy did not want to go to horse shows anymore. By Troy staying lame, they didn't have to. Brilliant!

She had never admitted this to herself, because she was always such a team player; moreover, they both had a secondary gain, because every weekend they had the barn to themselves, and Ava had an additional secondary gain: When she went to work and told everyone at lunchtime that she hadn't been able to go to the horse show, they all felt badly for her. She had been used to getting sympathy as a child when her parents divorced, so this was a familiar habit that she was happy to break.

We did a few rounds of tapping over the next week. Releasing all this old stuff gave Ava the confidence to still have fun at her barn when everyone else went to horse shows while she and Troy stayed home. She didn't need people to feel sorry for her at work anymore, and Troy was becoming more sound every day, with not a lame step.

The true test came when it was time for Troy to get a second set of X-rays following the diagnosis a couple of years earlier. The vet determined that this was the first time he had ever "undiagnosed" a horse with navicular disease.

Lily and Paralysis

Lily was a darling pug who was soulful, feisty, yet had an unmistakable inner diva that didn't hesitate to come out. Lily's biggest challenge was not just aging but degeneration in her spine, and her hind end had given out on her several times. Many veterinarians had told her human, Betsy, it was time to let Lily go.

Lily was Betsy's soul mate dog, so it did not feel like time to her. Her bouncy household also consisted of two much younger dogs, a Labrador and another very young Pug. To top it off, she was a vet technician, so there was a real part of her that struggled with the Western medicine answer to Lily's occasional paralysis.

We applied all of the healing methods I had to offer, along with those of other practitioners who would stop by my healing center. Eventually, I suggested EFT.

We tapped on Lily and Betsy around the fear and sadness of the diagnosis and would move to accepting miracles, regardless of what Western medical wisdom said.

I'm happy to report that Lily lasted another two and a half years, and most of it was still as a diva, feisty, and always soulful.

Cappuccino and Asthma

Cappuccino, a beautiful, 23-year-old Thoroughbred mare, came to stay at my center as a last-ditch effort to improve her worsening asthma. The dampness in the Seattle area was too much for Cappuccino. Not only were the medications not working but some were backfiring, giving her hives, or upsetting her tummy to the point of mild colic symptoms.

Amy, her person, had raised Cappuccino since birth, but had decided it would be best for Cappuccino's health for her to go into retirement in Arizona. To retire a beloved 23-year-old horse several states away seemed impossible, but if that would make the horse comfortable, Amy was willing to do it. After using all of my energetic techniques for the asthma, and knowing there would be a trailer in the next few days to pick up Cappuccino and take her to Arizona, I finally looked at Amy and said, "Let's tap."

Even though I had done animal communication, it was the channeling involved with tapping that revealed the big story. Amy "owned" another horse she didn't ride, and someone else was showing this super-fancy horse. Cappuccino was never going to go to a horse show. She wasn't that kind of girl. She was the down-home best friend who says, "Let's go on the trail." She felt tossed aside because of this fancy dude that Amy "part-owned."

Once this was released in both Amy and Cappuccino through tapping, they let out a sigh of relief that could have been felt in Arizona. Cappuccino never moved to Arizona. She stayed with Amy in Seattle until the day she died, about seven or eight years later. She never had an asthmatic attack again.

Star Wars and Lung Cancer

Occasionally, people brought cats to my healing center. Typically, with most cats, I either went to them or spent several days on the phone (before Zoom) connecting remotely around the world.

Star Wars was more of a doglike cat and didn't mind the adventure of traveling to me. He would walk around my place, smell the smells, then lay down on a dog bed for his work to be done.

Star Wars had been diagnosed with lung cancer, but in my medical intuition scans it seemed mild, almost lighter in his lungs than Cappuccino's asthma had felt. Still, he wasn't thriving, and this was partly why his person, Maria, brought him over for weekly proactive healing sessions with me.

Star Wars was so aloof, he had never revealed much in animal communication sessions before the healing, but after a couple of sessions, I asked Maria, "Did he lose a brother?" (I not only had a sense of this but also he reminded me of a cat called Spencer in Florida, so I couldn't resist asking.)

Maria nearly burst into tears and said, "Yes, he died so young, only three, and I'm not ready to lose Star Wars."

I tapped with each of them about the loss and grief, and did an extra round of tapping with Maria around her expectation that she would lose him.

Star Wars lived with lung cancer for a couple of years. She did eventually lose him, but it was like he had never been diagnosed. They were able to enjoy a normal life together.

Breaking It Down Emotionally

Health challenges often remind both human and animal of previous losses and the struggle to keep that beloved being alive.

For the animal, there are often amazing secondary gains, such as getting more attention, extra food, extra love, extra time in the car, extra one-on-one time, and so on. For the human, there is often a struggle with guilt and this potential loss reminding them of another loss, feeling like a failure, feeling out of control, and deep, deep despair.

In focusing on a perfect-world ending when doing tapping, it is important to dream—to see the miracle, to stretch toward it and say it out loud, and not only say it out loud but create a visionary/guided meditation for the animal companion to participate with you in the dream.

NOTE: For a sample tapping session template, please refer to Let's Tap in Chapter 5 and the Appendix.

9

End of Life

The short life span of our animals is just not fair. No matter how long the disease and dying process is or how prepared we think we are, there is never enough time. Time becomes everything. As our animals get older, or if we are in that dying stage with a beloved, it is definitely time to slow down and take our time.

In my *TEDx* talk, "Rainbow Bridge: Animals in Transition," I introduce the idea of Preciousville:

Meanwhile, in Preciousville, we slowed down time and noticed each other. We made up for each other's weaknesses in our older age. We laughed out loud at cats getting dogs to run through the house. We applauded a great dog trick. I rode my horses, even in the rain. We stretched time in that, this would never be again, like this. We were all for one and one for all. We were big love. Sure there were dog snarls, cat screeches and horse squeals . . . and human cussing . . . but those were momentary blips on the harmony screen.

Living with as many animals as I do (three horses, three dogs, and four cats), Preciousville could be a full time job! But even when animals aren't older or in a dying process, I do like to stay in Preciousville all the time . . . because we just don't know.

When we get out of "busy" and into this slowed-down state, we notice that our lives are always in some state of transition. Whether it's a job promotion, a lifestyle change, a new lover, a marriage evolving to the next level, a kid moving out, a series we are binge-watching, remodeling the kitchen—there are little transitions all day, every day, for us.

Yet, our animals depend on us for both that enrichment and stability. Even in times when we aren't in a death or dying stage, this concept of enjoying the moment with them in Preciousville could be employed the moment they move into our homes, and then this awareness of noticing becomes a habit. Everything becomes so beautiful those last months, those last moments when they are between worlds—painful but beautiful.

As I did while in practice as an animal communicator, and as I teach in my Animals in Transition courses, I am honored to hold space for people as they just grieve. There's nothing to say. It's not my place to make them feel better. They just get to be in that space.

That space is not always safe for them. They often hear from friends, "It's just a dog" or "It's just a cat," or "You can get another parakeet," and not even an acknowledgment that they have just lost a precious family member.

We often love animals with a purity of spirit. We are returned to our own pure spirit every time we gaze into their eyes. There aren't the complications we have with humans. That is why, often the loss is unbearable. The loss is so big, it seems like an empty cavern, because their love for their animal was so great.

I know, I'm making it all sound like it is some beautiful experience and you get a soundtrack with harps playing in the background. The truth is, it is gut-wrenchingly painful. What you do get is ugly-crying, puffy eyes, or worse, numbness. There is often a great amount of guilt accompanying grief. Plenty of times, there is regret. And there is fear—fear of losing, fear of pain, fear of dying.

So many New Age groups subscribe to the idea that it is easy for animals to transition. If that were true, they would slip out of their dog/cat/horse suits effortlessly. Nobody would fight, nobody would struggle. Yes, there are some animals that are evolved in their spirit around the concept of crossing the veil, and certainly, the hope is that we are all "ready" when the time comes. But it is as individual as it is with humans: some humans are ready, and others fear they didn't complete their business.

It is therefore our duty to check in with our animals about how they feel and how they feel about the others around them in order to support completion. Even then, they still may be afraid and may still have karma and contracts to work through. It is a process, a labor into the next world. It is not any easier for them than it is for us. In a perfect world, the process helps all of us get ready.

Fear of Letting Go

Duchess

Duchess was a 16-year-old cat who was in the advanced stages of cancer. Like her name, she was a classy cat and had dignity. She was holding steady and not getting markedly better or worse.

Her person, I.D., was so sad and was not ready to let her go. For I.D., Duchess represented a whole chapter in I.D.'s life, and she didn't know how she would manage without her beloved cat. I.D. left the corporate world to pursue a career in energy healing and felt the support from her cat, something she didn't necessarily get from other humans.

Upon checking in with Duchess in the animal communication and EFT investigation, she said that she was ready and comfortable with leaving. She shared that they had lost a cat many years before, Amadeus. Duchess remembered that I.D. was devastated by the loss of Amadeus and would be equally overcome with grief upon her own death.

Duchess also shared that I.D. had a young cat named Timothy, who was the polar opposite of Duchess. She felt his shenanigans would at least be entertaining. She also felt that I.D. was feeling abandoned. Duchess hated disappointing them.

When I did the EFT tapping just for Duchess, we reviewed all those feelings and emphasized the "I'm ready to go" and that she didn't want I.D. to worry so much.

After the tapping, I.D. had tears of relief rather than sadness and said that she was ready for Duchess to go. Duchess had a peaceful passing not long after that. I.D. was forever grateful for that shift.

Yogi

Wendy's soul mate horse Yogi has helped her build, run, and maintain her reiki school. Their communication has been so deep over the years that he once summoned her back from a trip. She was starting to feel like she was not in the moment with Yogi anymore, though, because she worried about the end of his life.

Julie is one of CWALU's graduates and teachers and is also a Lutheran minister. Counseling at this deep level is like a well-worn coat for her. She worked with Wendy and Yogi for animal communication and discovered that Yogi could feel her fear and was stern with her. It was getting in the way of their relationship. Wendy was not enjoying the remaining time with him and not seeing the health and strength he does have. Julie suggested EFT.

Julie tapped on Wendy feeling sad about being without Yogi: "Without taking care of him, who am I?" and "I want us both to be ready. I want us to stay connected." It was at this point that the tapping shifted to: "I have this relationship with Yogi. He is unstoppable, and death is not going to stop Yogi—this relationship we have is so strong it will continue." The tapping then wound down into a meditation with the wisdom circle to support them.

Now they just move into new phases of relationship together. She has accepted that he is both head and master teacher at her reiki school and gets to direct things. He is not retired. It's a new phase of ministry.

Grief for Humans and Animals

Penny

One of the graduates of my program, Ayat, is a seasoned foster person. She has a big heart for her fosters but knows that if she keeps one, that's one more dog that doesn't get a foster home.

Penny was not an easy dog to foster. She was not safe in her own skin and shut down. Ayat had to carry her downstairs, could not use the vacuum cleaner, and Penny was reactive around strangers and had high anxiety. At some point, Penny had been kicked, and even though her ribs had healed and Ayat could pick her up, she reacted to her sides being touched.

Through the investigation process, we discovered that Penny had been with a lady who had died and the woman's nephew had locked her out on a patio. Her anxiety was deep-seated and derived from this core grief—so simple, yet so complicated and sad. Even though Penny had experienced some painful things in life, she was a true caretaker and had been deeply loved. This was all gone now.

We tapped for a long time on the grief and feeling sad. We ended with "I am safe in my own skin." There is no doubt in my mind that the EFT helped immensely. Penny is a different dog now. She still has quirks! I also think the investigation process helped Penny be seen and heard for the first time since her person died.

Leo

Leo was a Shetland sheepdog, devoted not only to Marcia and her husband but had been an emotional support to many patients during Marcia's career as a therapist, angel guide, and shaman. When Leo was diagnosed with bone cancer, everyone was shattered. He was a ball of love, innocent yet wise and always there for others. Even though

Marcia has more tools than anyone to help with grief, she was unable to assuage her own. EFT offered her relief, as she unwound the story of seeing him limp, to shattering his knee, to finding out about his diagnosis, to the moment he passed.

We tapped on how devastated everyone felt: herself, her husband, the vets, and her clients. While Marcia was surrounded by others who shared the shock, grief, and loss, it didn't help one bit. The pain was too great. While tapping, we stayed on the shock of it all for several rounds and ended with finding peace in his passing.

Grief among the Animals

The physical act of separation from whether it is weaning animals, adopting out animals, or breaking up bonded pairs is a death. They will never see that litter mate, mother, father, pack mate, family member again.

Fancy

Over the years, I have talked to many of Barbara's horses as well as the horses she boards at her facility. She had a new horse I had not met before. This little horse, Fancy, seemed sweet yet had a melancholy sensibility to her. I was there to unlock whatever was going on with her, so I proceeded with the communication.

Within a few minutes, Fancy told me that she had "rock star" babies and started baring her teeth and pinning her ears at me in full protection mode, as if I were threatening her. I thought it was peculiar.

Barbara noticed and commented on how bizarre it was, saying, "She's so sweet. I've never seen her do anything like this."

I moved on with the communication, but Fancy wanted to continue protecting herself physically from me. When I relayed the information from Fancy to Barbara, Fancy really started swishing her tail in an agitated fashion, swinging her butt around in anticipation of a fight.

Barbara told me that Fancy had given birth to a dead foal and was immediately bred again. That second foal lived with her, side by side, for eight years and had recently been sold. Just like that, after eight years, her celebrated progeny, her beloved companion, was simply gone. When I realized that I had hit upon trapped grief, I thought EFT would really help.

I stood next to her shoulder to be out of striking range of her front feet, and certainly clear from her quickly swinging hind end. Because she was tied on either side of her halter, I knew she couldn't bite me. Then I started tapping.

I kept my tapping script simple, focusing on the loss and grief and how out of control life must seem. Within minutes, she was yawning and releasing and seemed much calmer. I tempted fate a bit and stepped away from her shoulder, and she was very peaceful and sweet.

Barbara couldn't believe her eyes. It was a seemingly spontaneous healing within minutes. The rest of my time with this lovely horse was very quiet. It was wonderful to see how willing she was to release this.

A couple of days later, I heard from Barbara, who reported: "Fancy is way more at ease, and her huge release of anger and grief is very apparent in her behavior and the energy everyone feels from her. Thank you for coming out and sharing your wonderful gift with us."

Zena

Zena was crestfallen after her beloved life partner, King, died. Both Zena and King were noble German Shepherds. King was eight when he died too early, and Zena was only five. How could she go on without him?

Her human, Katie, was equally bereft, as she shared a deep love for him as well. Katie felt as though King was a better soul mate than her husband! The pain was unfathomable, and it had been months. The once bouncy Zena was confused, mopey, and lethargic. Zena had always had King to look up to and didn't know how to navigate life without him.

After all of this was revealed in an animal communication session, we started EFT on Zena. She was stoic through the whole thing, and I had to trust that I had moved the needle on her grief. I moved on to tap with Katie. After her round of EFT, Katie felt much better, much lighter, and was grateful for the shift.

The next morning, I received a video of Zena doing zoomies in the backyard. She literally sprang back to life after months of being nearly nonresponsive. Zena never looked back. Her grief was complete.

Breaking It Down

When we investigate end of life or transitioning on behalf of the human, often we will find big feelings, such as guilt, worry, sadness, shock, feeling out of control, abandonment, and deep grief. It can often remind them of someone else's death that was untimely or couldn't be helped, therefore compounding this loss. In which case, it is valuable to sort out all the past and present feelings so the person can be truly present for this being.

In the animal's case, when doing the investigation, you will also find sadness, shock, feeling out of control and deep grief. You may also find that they worry for their human or other animals they are leaving behind.

NOTE: For a sample tapping session template, please refer to Let's Tap in Chapter 5 and the Appendix.

10

Gaining Experience in Real-World Practice

N ow that you have mastered the crazy hand movements with all of the points while saying words, did it work? Like I said before, it may have taken a while to develop the challenge the animal is facing, and it may take a while to undo it. Know that even if your animal is just starting to take a breath before reacting or taking a lighter step or you aren't as frustrated over the situation, this is progress and all part of the process.

How to Tell If the Work Is Complete

Obviously, a full-on miracle is a tell-tale sign that all is well. Short of that, watching for the baby steps and filling the void so to speak is what must happen.

When I say "filling the void," what I mean is that we want a replacement behavior for what was missing.

For example, say that normally on a walk, if I was not paying attention and my dog was leash-reactive, I would also go into reactivity. Now everyone is reactive, and we are lucky we get down the street.

The replacement behavior would be having the dog continually checking in with me, knowing that I'm coming around the corner and that barky Dalmatian is going to be at the fence line waiting for the entertainment of my dog losing it, and the big reward of a release as we walk on by and neither I nor my dog is reacting.

We must trust the process. My dog Delilah was a quick processor, and in the time it took for me to try to imagine she could change, she had already changed. Thankfully, Delilah is a fiery Sagittarius! I have other animals (mostly Taurus and Cancer) that wouldn't be that energetically mutable. They need to hang onto their story a little longer and chew on the idea that they really meant what they said when they vowed to release the story. We are all different. While we must trust the process, we must also trust who our animal is and recognize and celebrate how they process, and involves learning to honor how we process as well.

Tonight, I called a student who had asked the school's Facebook group for healing and/or prayers for her horse, which had a high fever due to an infected leg.

When I spoke to her, she said she had been using EFT on herself and that she had noticed a difference in how she responded. She wasn't panicked. She wasn't ready to load her horse into the trailer to get him to the hospital. Rather, she was calmly going to the store to get apple sauce to make his medications yummier.

She was grateful for this change in herself. I've been through some pretty big things with her, and I too am grateful for this shift! I'm happy to add that while it took a few days, the infection in the leg resolved.

When you've been tapping on yourself for a while, you will notice that everything around you has changed, when, in fact, it was you all along!

Behavioral Backslides

A backslide in behavior "feels like" the animal has gone back to the beginning and nothing has changed.

It is a great time for reflection, as a backslide is similar to what is considered a "healing crisis," so make sure to read on to the next section.

That said, a backslide offers an opportunity to review the eight steps:

1. Wow, we came far briefly!
2. What were all the steps we took in addition to tapping?
3. Did we fall back into an old mindset?
4. Did we fall back into old patterns/habits?
5. Is there something new to tap on here?
6. Is there something new that I could do that would elevate my emotional leadership?
7. Is there an outside circumstance contributing to this that I could either eliminate or work around?
8. How would I summarize what happened here?

When we ponder what our animal has been through to begin with then add that list of questions, we usually gain the compassion to go back to the drawing board and find our way through the situation. Usually

(I'm not saying always), we have not gone backward, but have hit a plateau and it is a "let's review" period.

How to Handle a Sudden Healing Crisis

If you have a condition and suddenly take 9,000 herbs to clear it or have an injury and get a massage, your body has to take the time to assimilate. This is called a "healing crisis."

If your body has been going along at a certain level with a disease and/or condition and you add something to "fix it," it may be in shock and say to you, "Hold the phone! What is all this comfrey for?"

Eventually the healing modality/technology/remedy settles in and is able to do its job, but even the healthiest of remedies can be a jolt to a system that has been used to its own status quo. Ultimately, a healing crisis is an opportunity for the body to detox and allow the true and deep healing to take place.

Like the behavioral backslide, while I was dealing with worsening symptoms, I would take the time to acknowledge and examine the eight steps listed above.

When to Repeat Treatments and How to Tweak the Script

I'm a believer in allowing things to settle in. I like to give things a few days, maybe even a week, because processing has a timeline of its own. But if I have a big challenge then I'm going to tap every day. It depends on the situation.

In my school, we have an outreach program for rescues/shelters with unadoptable animals. These animals get a communication with my advanced students and then someone is assigned to tap with the animal, if need be. In those cases, the animals are worked with every day for a few days. The rescue or shelter then arranges for training, so that new neural pathways are created and settle and the animal has a chance of getting adopted.

The script should shift from session to session, unless you feel as though the animal or human is too guarded. It is worth reviewing the investigation each time because some of the big emotions may have changed or other memories come up after the first tapping. It is also a good idea to take notes of where you noticed the animal really shifting during the tapping and see if that is reflected in real life.

For example, the other day I used EFT with a dog that has neurological symptoms and some other quirks. He wouldn't go up any stairs and was really stuck in some OCD patterns. While I was tapping with him, he was going along with it until I said "I'm really scared," and he tried to leave the room. I stayed with the emotion, and we moved through it. (You can actually watch this video on my YouTube channel.)

Since then, he can run up and down stairs and isn't as scared. This next tapping session, I will probably go into more of the disconnect in his physical body, because I feel like we cleared a lot of the overriding fear in that one session.

Conclusion

I hope this book has helped you and your animal companion(s). I know it helps me, my dogs, my cats, and my horses daily. I also see it move mountains with my students, clients, and teachers at CWALU.

It is an exciting time to be part of what I hope will become a movement, and I ask you to read along and hold a vision with me for this work and the animals around the world.

This movement involves defining new "family values." By that, I mean that our animal companions are family. We help instill these family values in others by leading by example, including acting as a supportive global village that, if it detects an ounce of willingness on the part of the human struggling with their animal's behavior, wellness, or relationship issues, has the tools and resources to help them out.

This movement has so many helpful tools and options that we are creating a "disposable-free zone," meaning that returning or owner-surrendering an animal to the rescue or shelter is never an option. If for some unforeseen reason the animal can't stay in the home, a safe landing with love and adoration is created as the outcome.

EFT is particularly helpful in the rescue and shelter communities, and I now have countless stories of animals that were adopted right after a round or two of EFT—animals that until then had been "tough to place."

The truth is, these animals are tough to place because they are a shell of their former selves, who they truly are, and we are not reading them correctly. They didn't work out somewhere and were left behind. They are grieving hard, the decision was completely out of their control, they have shut down emotionally, and then they don't seem adoptable. When I think of the staggering number of animals euthanized in this country, I believe we have genocide on our hands.

I hold a dream with my students that we could empty the cages. I ask you to join me in this vision. We can empty the shelters. The physical buildings where the shelters once were could become doggy

daycare centers, kennels, dog training centers, EFT for Animals educa-
tion centers, or cat grooming centers (okay, I'm kidding about the cat
grooming centers . . . maybe).

Then we could go to other countries where animals aren't valued
as much and start educating on compassion for animals and different
levels of care and/or we can bring their animals back to our empty
shelters because we will need animals to adopt out.

We could help the transition of animals used in laboratory testing
into homes where they are loved and adored. Traumatized animals
rescued from factory farms will live out their days in a beautiful sanc-
tuary and have their transition eased by EFT.

Wildlife, our not-so-distant cousins, are also family. Helping the
victims of poaching, habitat loss, hunting, and/or human wildlife
conflict will release the trauma through EFT. And of course, EFT
will also help humans entrenched in this work who are experiencing
"compassion fatigue."

You can see that there is no end to where this work can go. It is
much needed to release the suffering of the animals and the empathic
human souls who lament over their well-being. I hope you'll join me
in holding the vision.

Appendix

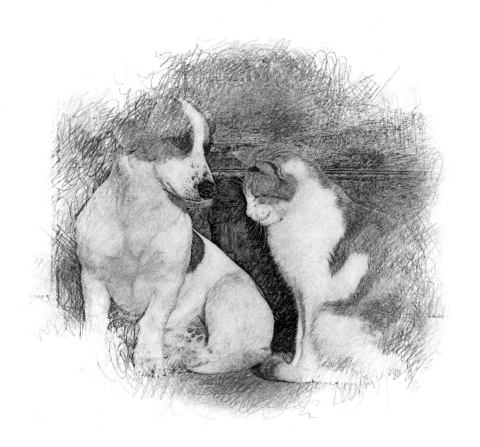

Tapping Template and Sample Scripts

The following is how I like to get started with tapping (see Chapter 5). Feel free to use this template for reference and personal use.

Grounding

Personally, I meditate daily and have a practice of using my other favorite technique, the Scalar Wave, on myself to ground my energy first thing in the morning. If I am tapping on an animal in person, I like to help them get grounded as well. I may just sit and take some deep breaths with them to calm them and try to match our breathing.

I might do something called the Bladder Sweep, which is a physical sweep down the bladder meridian. As we know from the first tapping point on the face, that is Bladder 1, the start of the Bladder meridian. It runs parallel to the spine, down the hind legs to the outside toe on both hind legs. I would stroke three times from the top of their head down to the left hind outside toe, then three times from the top of their head down to the right outside toe, then three times from the top of the head to the end of the tail. If they are missing a limb or the tail, I still do it to the phantom limb or tail.

Review

I like to review what the circumstances are, whether it is a relationship dynamic or an event that is causing the present reality.

I take the script (see farther down) and investigate *my own feelings (or those of the human I'm working with)* and take copious notes. While there may be a story as a framework for the situation, these notes largely identify several feelings and emotions involved in the current state. I take the script and investigate *the animal's feelings* based on either an animal communication session or what would very clearly be the feelings for the animal based on behavior, and again take copious notes. While there may be a story as a framework for the situation, these notes largely identify several feelings and emotions involved in the current state.

Intention

What is it I'm trying to accomplish here? What is my intention? Is it peace? Well-being? Getting clear on the intention is vital for a desired outcome.

Outcome

What is the final outcome? This is something worth spending time on at the end of the tapping, either by tapping several rounds or creating a visualization for you and your animal of the desired outcome for both (or all) beings. Even if the animal is going to transition (to a new home, a new job or the eternal home) have a peaceful vision like a guided meditation that you are able to say out loud and feel the joy, peace or relief that this can offer. All beings want safety and security above all else. Ending with the animal feeling safe, confident and feeling good in their own skin is also a wonderful outcome.

Sample Scripts

Please note, the following are sample scripts you can use to fill in the blanks. None of these points are necessarily connected to these specific parts of the script. Meaning, if you find an emotion that is triggered, or if you feel like the animal or human is not moving on a specific emotion, please tap several rounds of all of the points on the specific emotion. It is not about the story or the specific placement of the tapping points, it is about the emotion being released.

For more sample scripts and video demos please go to:
www.eftanimalsbook.com.

Sample Script – Investigation for the Human

Karate Chop point setup statement:

- *Round 1*: Share the story of what happened and your emotions around the experience, and end with "And I love and accept myself."
- *Round 2*: Share more of your story and your big emotions around the event or relationship, and end with "And I fully accept myself."
- *Round 3*: Share how this animal's big emotions continue to trigger you and end with "I honor the choices I'm making."

Inside eye socket: *When this happened* ....

....

OR

When my animal ....

Outside eye socket: *I feel* ....

....

Under eye: *I also feel* ....

....

Under nose: *I continue to feel* ....

....

Chin: *People around me think* ....

....

Collarbone: *Which makes me feel even more* ....

....

Pick one of the following:

Top of head: *If I'm honest, I may be getting a secondary gain of* ....

....

It's familiar and reminds me of..

Pick one of the following transition setups:

Inside eye socket: *I am feeling blocked/resistant to shift/I'm in a big battle because* ....

....

....

I struggle with my deep-seated belief/vow/loyalty to my feelings,

because ....

....

Big Forgiveness or Letting-Go Transition Statement

Pick one of the following:

Outside eye socket: *I forgive myself. I am ready to let this go.*

It's time to move on.

I'm ready to try something new.

I can't take it anymore.

Under eye: *In a perfect world my animal companion would* ....

....

....

Under nose: *And we would feel* ....

....

....

NOTE: If a big feeling doesn't seem to release, don't hesitate to tap several rounds (through all of the points) just on that one emotion or feeling.

Sample Script – Investigation for the Animal

Inside eye socket: *When I feel* ....

....

OR

when .... *happens*

Outside eye socket: *I feel* ....

....

Under the eye: *I also feel* ....

Top of the nose: *I continue to feel* ....

....

Under the chin: *People around me think* ....

....

Collarbone: *Which makes me feel even more* ....

....

Pick one of the following:

Top of head: *If I'm honest, I may be getting a secondary gain of* ....

....

....

It's familiar and reminds me of ....

....

Pick one of the following:

Top of head: *If I'm honest, I may be getting a secondary gain of* ....

....

It's familiar and reminds me of ....

....

Pick one of the following:

Top of head: *If I'm honest, I may be getting a secondary gain of* ....

....

It's familiar and reminds me of..

....

Pick one of the following transition setups:

Inside the eye socket: *I am feeling blocked/resistant to shift/I'm in a big battle, because* ....

....

I struggle with my deep-seated belief/vow/loyalty to my feelings, because

....

Big Forgiveness or Letting-Go Transition Statement

Pick one of the following:

Outside eye socket: *I forgive myself. I am ready to let this go (statement can be reversed).*

It's time to move on.

I'm ready to try something new.

I can't take it anymore.

Top of the nose: *In a perfect world my person and I would* ....

....

Under the chin: *And we would feel* ....

....

NOTE: If a big feeling doesn't seem to release, don't hesitate to tap several rounds (through all of the points) just on that one emotion or feeling.

Bibliography

Bekoff, Mark. *The Emotional Lives of Animals: A Leading Scientist Explores Animal Joy, Sorrow and Empathy – and Why They Matter*. San Francisco, CA: New World Library, 2010.

Levine, Peter. *Waking the Tiger: Healing Trauma*. Illustrated edition. Berkeley, CA: North Atlantic Books, 1997.

Panksepp, Jaak. *Affective Neuroscience: The Foundations of Human and Animal Emotions*. New York: Oxford University Press, 1998.

Ranquet, Joan. *Communication with All Life: Revelations of an Animal Communicator*. Carlsbad, CA: Hay House, 2015.

_____. *Energy Healing for Animals: A Hands-On Guide For Enhancing the Health, Longevity and Happiness of Your Pets*. Louisville, CO: Sounds True, 2015.

Acknowledgments

I am so grateful for all the people that have taken a risk and let me try this weird "tapping thing" on their animal. All those experiences, however small or giant and impactful, are what created this volume of work. I am full of gratitude for all the clients that, over the last 30 or so years, have helped me develop and blossom as an animal communicator and healer.

I am grateful to all the students and teachers at the school I founded, Communication with all Life University (CWALU), as well as the support team that props up CWALU daily. The school is made better by its many associations with sanctuaries, centers, rescues, and shelters. Thank you all!

I am grateful to Sabine Weeke and Findhorn Press. This wouldn't have been possible without my dear friend Margaret Ann Lembo. Thank you, Margaret!

My animals have put up with a lot of boredom, as I have been typing for days, it seems. I want to thank them for their patience. And I am grateful to my friends and inner circle for their support and cheerleading.

I have a feeling that there is a celebration among my animals that are hanging out at the Rainbow Bridge, and my parents have joined them.

About the Author

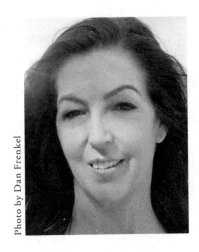

Photo by Dan Frenkel

Joan Ranquet is an inspired animal communicator, energy healer, and educator. The founder of the Communication with All Life University (CWALU), a certification program for animal communication and energy healing, she teaches through workshops, wildlife retreats, and private sessions.

Passionate about animals all her life, Joan is the author of two books: *Communication with All Life* and *Energy Healing for Animals*. Her TEDx talk, "The Rainbow Bridge: Animals in Transition," received over 306,000 views on YouTube. It's no surprise that MSN (Microsoft Network) has deemed her one of the "Top 25 People Who Do What They Love."

Joan lives in Santa Clarita, California, with her three horses, three dogs, and four cats.

For further information visit: **https://joanranquet.com**.

FINDHORN PRESS

Life-Changing Books

Learn more about us and our books at
www.findhornpress.com

For information on the Findhorn Foundation:
www.findhorn.org